In Her Own Voice

IN HER OWN VOICE

Childbirth Stories from Mennonite Women

Collected, edited, and translated by
Katherine Martens
and Heidi Harms

With a foreword by
Joan Thomas

for Willie - thanks so much for coming! Heidi 9-May-97
Katherine

THE UNIVERSITY OF MANITOBA PRESS

Printed in Canada

Printed on recycled, acid-free paper ∞

Cover photograph courtesy Erica Ens

Design: eye-to-eye design

Canadian Cataloguing in Publication Data

Martens, Katherine, 1935-

In her own voice

Includes bibliographical references.

ISBN 0-88755-642-6

1. Mennonite women – Manitoba – Interviews.
2. Childbirth – Manitoba. 3. Birth customs – Manitoba.
4. Mothers – Manitoba – Interviews. I. Harms, Heidi, 1953-
II. Title

RG560.M37 1997 392.1'2'088287 C97-920040-7

The publisher gratefully acknowledges the support for its publishing program provided by the Manitoba Arts Council and the Manitoba Department of Culture, Heritage and Citizenship.

Contents

Foreword

THE STORIES OF HOW WE GIVE BIRTH are among the most joyous and momentous stories we have, but until recently they have been held in the hearts of women. It's so very hard to put into words what being pregnant and bearing a child is like — that sense of one's body being taken over by forces that are unfamiliar and powerful yet nevertheless our own, those feelings of terror and anticipation, pain and pleasure mixed in unparalleled intensity. When I read, in this volume of birth stories, Maria Reimer's translation of the Low German expression for being pregnant — "being in the other time" — I felt a throb of recognition. For many women, becoming mothers is the ultimate transforming experience, changing us in ways that we could not have imagined. It's an experience that is hard to articulate, but as human beings we do grapple with the hard-to-tell stories. Those other transformational experiences — sex and death — are at the heart of many of our oral stories and most of our literature. The narratives we tell are our way of making meaning of our experience. They reflect who we are, and they shape us. What is significant about our stories of giving birth is that we have so few of them. There is a silence around childbirth that we are all familiar with: the sudden drop of voices in the kitchen when women talk alone, the outlandish stories told to children to explain the arrival of a new baby.

There are no doubt many reasons for this. If sex and death are hard to talk about, childbirth carries associations of both. The possibility of dying in childbirth was very real for women of our grandparents' generation. Even in normal labour and delivery, there is a sense of moving into the unknown that some of the women in these pages associate with death. And pregnancy is sexuality made manifest, sexuality in very female terms, a confrontation with our biology. Before having a child, we contemplate the cycle of life and death in existential terms, and we wonder at the mystery of it. After, we know about it in our bodies rather than our heads; we have been drawn in — into our bodies in a new way, as well as into the cycle. But for society, the fact that birth stories centre in women's bodies presents a problem. A centuries-old societal shame and fear is triggered. I've heard the sanction against talking about childbirth openly expressed as a need to protect men and their sexual interest in their wives: a man should never know what his wife went through in childbirth or he would never touch her again.

I wonder to what extent our attitude to childbirth in the Western world is still affected by the Old Testament curse that women should give birth in pain. If childbearing is our lot in life — our punishment, even, for a sin that is vaguely equated with being female — talking about it brings up the shadow of that sin. Anna Fullerton, one of the women whose stories appears here, remembers, "Later I would talk about it, and people seemed to think there was something the matter with me." Maybe because this prohibition was broken only for the exceptional stories, the ones told in low voices in the kitchen, there is the assumption that birth stories will be "horror stories."

We have a long history of not telling, then, which becomes a kind of forgetting. When I was pregnant and longing to hear about the experiences of women older than I was, I felt that I was coming up against a collective amnesia about giving birth. Amnesia was in fact a reality for many women of my grandmother's and mother's generation, who were administered amnesia-inducing drugs during labour and delivery — from Twilight Sleep in the 1920s (a mixture of morphine and scopolamine) to Paraldehyde and Nembutal through the forties and fifties. I hear about these drugs with something approaching horror: horror that a woman should feel all the pain of her contractions, but be disoriented, confused, unable to work with her labour, that she should in consequence need to be "restrained," and that she should remember nothing of the birth of her child.

Our silence about childbirth is ending, as anyone who has been pregnant within the last fifteen years will know. I remember coming home from social events before my daughter was born, reeling with the recounted experiences of friends and acquaintances and complete strangers. What I heard were usually anecdotes — ritualized, reduced. I was amazed at the matter-of-fact tone of many of the women who talked to me. Their stories *had* become matters of fact, all of the wonder and terror falling away. As a society we're in a transition stage: the medical details of childbirth are the subject of open discussions, but there are very few situations where the whole story can be told.

The value of *In Her Own Voice* is that it creates one of those situations. Katherine Martens has given the women she interviewed the opportunity to remember, and a warm and accepting environment where it was possible to reflect on the meaning of those memories. Heidi Harms's skill as translator and transcriber, and the respect with which she viewed these oral histories, is apparent in the way that individual personalities and voices emerge from the pages of *In Her Own Voice.*

These stories put the experience of birthing in the context of a woman's whole life. Gertrude Epp's childbirth experiences are part of a bigger story of being separated from her family and adjusting to a new country. Marjorie Martin's experience of giving birth is told, as it needs to be, in the context of the adoption of her first two children and the death of her oldest daughter. And the stories in this volume are not horror stories. They are, by Katherine Martens's deliberate decision, not exceptional stories in the usual sense of the word; the premise of *In Her Own Voice* is that there is enough meaning in every birth, as in every death, to warrant the telling. There are funny stories here (I recall the moment in Margaret Sawatzky's story when the lamp began to sway as Margaret's husband, who was holding it, gradually succumbed to chloroform), there is drama, and there is the remembered delight of having an infant fall asleep at the breast.

Katherine Martens interviewed women from three generations. Their childbirth experiences represent three distinct stages in Western attitudes to childbirth. The first-stage interviews, those from the twenties and thirties, call us back to the times when preparations for childbirth included tearing up an old coverlet to make a cradle for the baby, and nailing the well shut so that the older children wouldn't fall in while their mother was occupied with her labour. In spite of the physical difficulties of life in a pioneer home, and the risks of possible complications without medical help, many of the older women interviewed here gave birth in circumstances that we now consider ideal: in a familiar setting, often with their own mother for support, sometimes with a midwife who brought her own children along and made soup and biscuits for family. As we move gradually back to a more natural way of childbirth, these stories from the early part of the century provide an important reference.

The stories of women who gave birth in the fifties, sixties, and seventies are all stories of hospital births, at a time when the medicalization of childbirth was at its height. What makes the strongest impression in these stories is not the natural difficulties of labour and delivery but a sense of imposed hardship: being isolated from close family members (including her husband), being denied a choice in how labour was managed, trying futilely to delay delivery until the arrival of the doctor, missing the first moments of a baby's life, enduring the pain of an infected episiotomy. These stories remind us that what hospitals might consider a routine labour and delivery may be remembered by women as a humiliating and terrifying experience.

Many of the stories of the younger mothers in this collection are stories of women reclaiming the birth process. They begin in general with a deliberate choice to have a child — sometimes still with the recognition of grave risks, as the stories of Sue Klassen and Robyn Epp remind us. These mothers often have a degree of information and choice that women have not had in the past, choices about where and how the birth will take place. Many of these contemporary women require a particular kind of courage: if they choose to exercise more control over the birth situation, they will be held responsible if something goes wrong. Though undoubtedly their highest priority is the safe arrival of a healthy baby, these are women who ask something of the birth experience.

The stories in *In Her Own Voice* represent the birth stories of all women in many respects. There are stories of having ten babies or having one, of Caesarean births, of adoption, of choosing to have a child as a single parent, of births that go as planned, and births that take everyone by surprise. Because the women interviewed are Mennonite women, this volume adds women's voices to existing histories of Mennonite communities. Maria Reimer's faith, her sense of partnership with God in creating a new life, is essential to her experience as a mother. Aggie Klassen's flight from Russia, Anna Fullerton's pain at being ostracized within her own family because she left the church, Peggy Regehr's struggle to have women's work valued in a Mennonite service organization — these experiences may be particular to the Mennonite community, but they have parallels in all our lives.

Taken together, these stories become a powerful collaborative voice. What I hear in them is something that hospitals have been slow to recognize: an understanding and acceptance of the fact that a natural process like childbirth is essentially uncontrollable, and women's strong desire that childbirth not be viewed as an unfortunate hurdle between themselves and motherhood, but as an enriching experience in itself. Katherine Martens's candid and courageous exploration of her own childbirth experiences sets the tone for this collection. Without beginning from a political premise, a politic emerges. It's there in the rueful comments of healthy women who were asked to stay in bed for ten days after giving birth, and it's there in other interviews in a clear recognition that the way we treat women giving birth is an expression of how we view women's value to our society. Peggy Regehr says, "Being in such a foggy state at something which is such an important part of a woman's life was an injustice to me as a woman."

This is the sort of female voice, both personal and collective, that I felt starved for when I was pregnant. Reading these stories, you may find yourself drawn back, as I did, into your own memories of childbirth, and feel the ache to talk about what those experiences meant. Katherine Martens was aware as she interviewed these women of the gift they were giving in telling their stories. What struck me also was the gift she and Heidi Harms gave each woman by creating a situation where the value of their stories would be recognized. This is so important, because eventually, for most of us, the memory becomes what is told.

Childbirth stories are revolutionary stories because they come out of silence, and because they change the way we see the experience of giving birth, helping us to revise a mythology of childbirth that was formed centuries ago. Margaret Laurence once recounted a reviewer's contemptuous reaction to the fact that she had included "the obligatory account of childbirth" in one of her novels. In one respect this reviewer was right. Birth stories *are* obligatory for a meaningful account of women's lives. The stories in *In Her Own Voice* provide one of the missing threads of our social narrative.

Joan Thomas

Acknowledgements

WITH THANKS TO: Ken Reddig, Centre for Mennonite Brethren Studies; Lawrence Klippenstein and Jim Suderman, Mennonite Heritage Centre; Jocelyn McKillop and Gilbert Comeault of the Provincial Archives of Manitoba, who gave support during the interview process; Manitoba Culture, Heritage and Citizenship, Oral History Grants Program; Canada Council Explorations Program; Manitoba Arts Council, for financial support; Darlene Birch and Anessa Maize, practising traditional midwives, and Anita Schroeder King, for stories and videos of homebirths; Di Brandt, who used seven interviews in her Ph.D. dissertation and thus introduced Heidi Harms as translator/transcriber and editor to the interviews; David Carr, Carol Dahlstrom, Allison Campbell of the University of Manitoba Press, who guided us through the book process; all the women who graciously gave their time and energy and talked so openly about so intimate a subject and gave permission for their interviews to be included.

INTRODUCTION

AT ONE TIME OR OTHER, all small children are curious about where babies come from. When I was four or five, I overheard my sisters talking about a woman who had just given birth. "Where do babies come from?" I asked. "From the Eaton's catalogue," one of my sisters replied, with just a hint of a smile. An image of the rows of babies in the catalogue advertisements for baby clothes flashed through my head. Then I had another thought. I had seen mail-order parcels from Eaton's sent back; "goods satisfactory or money refunded" was their guarantee. I was shocked. Could babies be sent back too?

Many years later, Mary Wall, a friend of my parents, told me another birth story. "When I was a little girl my father put my sister Tina and me into the sleigh on a cold winter day and took us to Gramma's for the night. He said a stork might come to the house. When I walked into the house the next day I saw no sign of Mother. I walked into my parents' bedroom and saw the cradle, usually stored in the attic, beside the bed in which my mother lay. It was unheard of for Mother to be in bed in the middle of the day. I tiptoed to the side of the cradle and saw a tiny baby. Children were not told a word about the event. That's the way it was done."

Mary's story fascinated me and stayed in the back of my mind. The curiosity about birth and birth giving had never left me, maybe because so few women ever talk about their birth experiences. In 1988, when the

Manitoba government announced a program to collect oral history interviews, I thought, Why not apply to interview women about their birth stories? I had gained some experience collecting interviews a few years earlier for a family memoir.

I decided to interview Mennonite women for several reasons. I was born and grew up in a Mennonite home in southern Manitoba, and although I left the Mennonite church when I was thirty, I still have many connections in the Mennonite community. I knew I would be finding women to interview by word of mouth, and thought it would be simplest if I looked within a group that was familiar to me. In fact, some older Mennonites feel most comfortable speaking German or Plautdietsch (the Mennonite dialect of Low German), and so by interviewing older Mennonite women in their own language I would be helping to preserve a part of Mennonite culture.

I had another reason for wanting to hear the stories of women. When I had interviewed a number of my father's colleagues for a family memoir, my mother asked, "What does she want from all these men?" I pondered that question. Our family life had revolved around my father and his work as a lay minister in the church. He had an important role in the community while my mother's role as wife and mother had lesser status. I decided that the next time I did a project about the Mennonite community, I would focus on women.

THE INTERVIEWS

During the twelve months when I was interviewing Mennonite women, I felt as if I were on a journey or quest. I began my interviews with a few questions, some fear, buried anger, and burning curiosity. Why did many of these women want to be "put out" for the birth of their babies? I wanted to hear from those whose lives were dominated by their role as mothers, who had up to fifteen children in years spanning the Depression. Childbirth happened in the midst of family and community life and in the context of other life events. Older women sometimes took the time to tell their whole life stories.

I wanted to hear the stories of mothers — my own mother and others. Often when I first approached a woman she said, "Oh, but I don't have any horror stories." Even more frequently I heard, "Why would you want to interview me? I don't have a story to tell." Mennonite women have been silent so long and have swallowed their thoughts and feelings so often, they are no longer aware of having anything worth saying.

The stories I heard during the twelve months evoked both joy and sadness. Childbirth is a time when our private and public lives intersect profoundly. I was not looking only for dramatic stories, but one was Helen

Wedel's description of a nurse pushing back her baby when she was in advanced labour to allow a doctor to deliver it. Similarly, Anna Thiessen's account of her hands being tied during childbirth was a painful reminder of a practice that continued into the sixties. Both Anna Fullerton and Margaret Sawatzky described how they watched the sunrise on a beautiful spring morning just prior to entering the hospital to give birth. The build-up of excitement and then the lyrical peace of home births are recounted from the mother's point of view by Sue Klassen, Evelyn Rempel Petkau, and Elizabeth Krahn, and from the perspective of a grandmother by Elsa Neufeld. Peggy Regehr tells of the transformation of a self-conscious young mother into an articulate older woman who struggles for fair treatment in her work with the Mennonite Central Committee. Di Brandt describes the shock of realizing that her academic studies were useless in terms of preparing her for maternity and in particular for the physical reality of pregnancy.

These accounts offer many different views of the experience of birth giving. Childbirth can be a transformative rite of passage. For many women it marked the passage to responsible adulthood. It could be an overwhelming experience. Maria Reimer remembered feelings of a close connection with God during the births of her children. She also recognized the association of childbirth with female support and solidarity; that is, she came to realize the value of female friends: "If only my husband could understand me better! But what can you expect from a man who has never been pregnant, or has never been a woman?" Agatha Warkentin credits her mother-in-law with much-needed support in the form of babysitting. Elsa Neufeld and Gertrude Epp, among others, tell stories of women who helped each other during childbirth. But childbirth is by no means an experience a woman must have. Magdalene Redekop and Marjorie Neufeld Martin talk eloquently about becoming mothers through adoption.

Nine of the women included in this book were born in the first two decades of this century. While these interviews were not intended to gather historical material, the lives of the women were touched by historical events. Some of the descendants of the 1870s wave of immigrants are Anna Thiessen, Sara Kroeker, Mrs. A, and Maria Reimer. Margaret Sawatzky, Helen Wedel, Gertrude Epp, and Agatha Martens came to Canada in the 1920s in the aftermath of the Russian Revolution. Gertrude, the oldest narrator, was pregnant during her voyage across the ocean, while Agatha's family came when she was only six and a half. Aggie Klassen, who narrowly escaped from Siberia during the Stalinist era, was part of the post-revolutionary 1940s immigration of Mennonites.

At first I intended to interview mostly older women, with perhaps a few younger ones for contrast. Primarily, I wanted to preserve the stories of these older women while it was still possible. Later on, as I began to have difficulty finding older women who would talk to me about childbirth, I turned to more women in their forties, thirties, and even twenties. These younger women, beginning with Elizabeth Krahn, changed the focus of the interviews from the past to the present. The young women, like their older counterparts, are struggling not merely to survive a rite of passage but to find dignity and meaning in the experience. Altogether, I interviewed forty-four women, twenty-six of whose edited interviews are included in this book. They cover a full range of ages and life experiences. The oldest narrator in this book, Gertrude Epp, was born in 1900, and the youngest, Roberta Loughrin, was born sixty-six years later.

These women also represent the full range of identification with the Mennonite community. Hildegard Martens, for instance, stopped attending the Mennonite church at age nineteen, and her only contact with Mennonites for the past three decades has been her immediate family and friends. By contrast, Maria Reimer lived all her life in a Mennonite community in southern Manitoba, was a devout church member and Christian, and could be said to be Mennonite through and through. Two narrators, Marjorie Neufeld Martin and Sue Klassen, are not Mennonites by birth.

Not everyone I approached wanted to relive her memories. After a preliminary interview, one woman cancelled our appointment for a taping. "My doctor says I shouldn't talk about things that depress me. After your visit I remembered how depressed I was during the years when I was having children." Another gave a lively pre-interview, in which she described the Russian Revolution and her flight to Canada. The night after our talk she had a dream in which her dead husband appeared and said, "Lot daut mau toch, Tin" ("Just leave that alone, Tina"). She, too, cancelled our taping session. One elderly woman declined to be interviewed because, in her words, "If I can't tell the whole truth I would rather not tell the story." The women who agreed to be taped, then, are not the silent ones but those who have made their peace with life and can talk about the past without overwhelming regret or pain.

My own goals changed as the interviews progressed. When I began, I saw my role as a skilled interviewer who would control and direct the sessions. After I had listened to the tape of my interview with Maria Reimer, who was then eighty-four years old and whose interview was my fifth, these ideas were thrown out the window. Her story took centre stage. It became my goal to find women who would tell their stories if I created the environment in which they could relate them. I began to see that my method was similar to that of a traditional lay midwife, which appealed to me. Like a midwife, I would be with a woman but would not necessarily intervene in her process. A midwife does not dictate the structure and form that the labour should take, but allows the woman to give birth in her own way and does not interfere unless she is asked for assistance. I did not intend to be coldly objective, but to be a living person who listened and responded to the story. The subject matter of these interviews just would not allow me to be objective. What could be more subjective than giving birth?

During the time I was interviewing these women, my mother's life was coming to an end. I spent hours at her bedside in the hospital. On one of these visits, she once again told me the story of my birth. It had been a late summer evening, and relatives had dropped in to visit. This would be my parents' first hospital birth, which meant that as soon as labour started they would have to begin the eighty-mile drive to the hospital in Winnipeg. Mother noticed she was in labour early in the evening but remained quiet while the guests stayed until late. After they had left, my father reproached her. "You hardly spoke to my relatives," he scolded. All she could say was, "We'd better leave for Winnipeg, because my time has come." They left immediately, and after a long and rough car ride I was born as soon as they arrived at Concordia Hospital in the wee hours of the morning. Later that day, as she brought me in to my mother, the nurse joked, "Mrs. Klassen, your baby girl has red bumps on her forehead. She wanted to be born sooner, but I guess you didn't want to have a baby in the car." When she told me the story this time, my mother mused that, of course, she could have been more assertive and insisted that Father take her to Winnipeg as soon as she felt her labour begin. She seemed surprised herself that she could interpret the story in a new way after all these years. The very act of telling her story gave her a new perspective.

As I listened to the stories of these mothers, I gradually became aware that all my life my own mother had been trying to tell me her life story in her own way, but that I had paid little attention. Her family stories always seemed so entangled. But now, when I started listening to her again, the stories began to hang together better. Her stories were like yarn, the strands twisted and turned, but what seemed to be digressions were merely strands that intertwined with the other strands. She was my first example of stream of consciousness in real life. "Now where was I?" she might say. Later, this was a question I often heard repeated by the women I interviewed.

MY FIRST BIRTH GIVING

Like the women I interviewed, I am a mother and have my own story. The events of my first birth giving had a strong effect on me and prompted me to find women who could answer questions I still had many years later. In

September 1962 I checked into a Toronto hospital to have my first baby. I passionately wanted to have a natural birth; that is, I did not want anesthesia and I wanted to do the breathing I had practised in prenatal classes. On entering the huge hospital I was overwhelmed by the strangeness of a place where I knew no one. At home my labour pains had been strong and frequent, but they became weaker and less frequent after I entered the hospital. How I needed a familiar face, a hand to hold, to be touched with tenderness; but not even my doctor was there, only his substitute. They told my husband to go home. The doctor came late at night and told me not to be a martyr: take the Demerol and try to get some sleep, and the baby would be born in good time. It sounded so easy. Morning came and he returned but I had no labour pains, and I was tired and discouraged. The drugs had stopped labour. The doctor ordered Pitocin to restart it.

Though it is easy to blame the doctor or the hospital, neither of them alone is at fault. What was I doing in a hospital when giving birth is not a disease but a natural process? Where were my mother and sisters? Where were the women who used to take care of the birthing mother? Why was I surrounded by strangers when birth is an intimate and sensual experience? What kind of culture strips women of all personal power and choice during a rite of passage in which they give life? The medical profession has for the past century had birthing women assume the worst possible position (lying supine), one that is unsafe for both mother and child, that is convenient for the doctor but not for the woman giving birth. My baby was delivered with forceps in the late afternoon after I had taken a drug to stimulate labour. He was brain damaged and lived fewer than twenty-four hours. After the autopsy they told us the baby had died as a result of difficulties during birth.

I returned to my room in the hospital knowing that my baby would live less than a day. A September thunder-and-lightning storm crashed outside my hospital window, breaking a late-summer heat wave. I remembered my mother saying thunder was God talking. I went to the window and said to the storm, "Stop shouting, and listen to me for a change. I put my faith in my doctors and what has it done for me? From now on I will trust myself." I never forgot those feelings. Before I gave birth in a modern hospital I thought I could reach my goals in life with good will and ladylike behaviour. The humiliation of being treated like a child while attempting to give birth like a man transformed me.

My first birth experience came back to haunt me in the anniversary year when my first baby would have been twenty-five years old. By then I had given birth to three healthy babies. During these births I had refused Demerol and insisted that my husband be with me. Yet I felt I had not finished what

I needed to do. When I began these interviews I knew I would be forced to immerse myself in stories of childbirth. I hoped that by confronting these stories and images directly I would finally resolve the anger and grief that still persisted from that first birth.

THE MENNONITES

Mennonites first came into existence in Germany, Switzerland, and the Netherlands during the sixteenth century and are named after one of their leaders, Menno Simons. As part of the left wing of the Reformation, they were Anabaptists who insisted on complete separation of church and state. A large number of Mennonites moved to the Vistula delta of Prussia where they became skilled at draining and farming flooded land. Beginning in 1774, there was a movement of Mennonites to Ukraine, where Catherine the Great invited them to settle on a vast tract of farmland. In the 1870s the first of these Mennonites (known as Kanadier) began to immigrate to the Canadian Prairies. They were attracted to a country where a monarch still ruled and where they were promised freedom of religion and education and exemption from military service. In the 1920s the next wave of Mennonite families (the Russländа) came, fleeing the Russian Revolution. A final group of immigrants came in the 1940s after the Second World War. The Mennonites built many communities in southern Manitoba, centred around towns such as Steinbach, Altona, and Winkler.

The Mennonite community seven miles north of Homewood, Manitoba, where I grew up, was a tiny enclave surrounded by "the English," as we referred to everyone who was not Mennonite. As schoolchildren we had no acquaintances who were not Mennonite. Even among Mennonites there were divisions — divisions among different groups of immigrants and among the many different church congregations: Mennonite Brethren, the Bergthaler (to which we belonged), Evangelical Mennonite Conference, Rudnerweider, Holdeman, and others. For us, each group had its place in the hierarchy. The English were on top, then the Russlända, then the Kanadier. When I was introduced to Anna Fullerton, I realized she was the first person with a Holdeman background whom I had ever met. We laughed when we compared ratings. She told me members of her church would have looked down on us Bergthalers. In their eyes we were worldly and not as pious as they. I would have looked down on her because the women in the Holdeman church wear a little head covering, a visible sign of being different.

Mennonites believe in the fellowship of believers, and that all believers have equal access to God, without the intercession of the clergy. Paradoxically, in practice this equality seems to be reserved for male church members. Their patriarchy is not different from patriarchy in other groups. In one Mennonite family I know, the father died a generation ago, leaving his wife and two unmarried children in their twenties. The son, much younger than his mother, took over the financial affairs of the farm. His sister, who was close to his age, ordered some goods from Eaton's catalogue without asking his permission, though she consulted her mother. He asserted his authority over her with physical punishment to demonstrate that he was now the head of the family. The myth was that men's work produced money and kept the economy going while women, with their foolish spending on amenities for the house, wasted money and made no material contribution to the household.

I learned to accept my father's statements because he had authority over me, my mother's because she had jurisdiction over the girls, my brothers' because they were older and they were men, my sisters' because they were older, my doctor's because he knew better than I what was good for me, and my husband's because he was in a scientific profession.

There is, of course, a healthy hierarchical ordering of the family in which the child knows the parents can be depended upon to provide an environment in which the children's needs are met, and where children have rights and responsibilities suitable to their age and maturity. When a mother's contribution to the household and family is recognized, a female child should have less conflict with regard to identification with her parents.

One way of ensuring conformity and asserting the authority of the Mennonite church is the practice of avoidance, or "shunning," which had its beginnings in the sixteenth century. While many branches of the Mennonite church have not practised shunning, or avoidance, since the beginning of the twentieth century, others, such as the Church of God in Christ (also known as the Holdeman church), held on to the practice. In the 1940s Anna Fullerton's father was shunned. To this day she does not know the reasons for this shunning, and her father may never have known either, since the church did not have to give a reason to initiate a shunning. When a member of the church is being shunned, other members will not associate with him or her; the member's own family may even refuse to eat with him or her at the table.

Women's place in Mennonite churches varies, depending on the congregation. The one I joined in my youth had "brotherhood" meetings, where male members met to discuss the business of the church. Women were not forbidden to attend, but neither were they encouraged. If she had a concern she wanted to bring forward, the wise woman told her husband to raise it. He might present it without enthusiasm or not at all because it was not his own idea, and she had no recourse. There was no scorn like the scorn for a man who was "henpecked," whose wife "wore the pants in the family."

In traditional Mennonite society, sex before marriage was sin, and, in marriage, refusing to have sex with one's husband was sin. Mennonites had large families; ten to sixteen children were not uncommon. These large families were a result of ignorance of birth control or the belief that such methods were sinful, not the result of a strong desire on the part of women to be pregnant every year. Some enlightened couples — perhaps primarily the immigrants who came in the 1920s — practised birth control, and since there is no confessional in the Mennonite church, they could not be reprimanded. When a woman wanted to use birth control but her husband strongly objected, could she abstain from sexual relations? An older woman I interviewed said she found herself in a dilemma. Saying yes to sex, she risked pregnancy, but the Bible told her that in refusing she was sinning by denying her husband his rights. My mother, who bore fifteen children, said she did not resent any of us, but she resented the fact that she had to bring us up alone. My father was both a farmer and a lay minister, and often Mother was left alone to cope with the farm and the children while Father was away on church business.

In the past, one characteristic of the Mennonite identity was the language, Plautdietsch, which is a form of Low German. For some of the older women interviewed here, Plautdietsch had been the language of daily life. Even when they speak English they retain some of the syntax and flavour of Plautdietsch. Examples are Anna Thiessen and Sara Kroeker. Children of my generation grew up speaking German or Plautdietsch at home. When I was in elementary school during the Second World War we were forbidden to speak German or Plautdietsch in school, or even outside the classroom during recess. Later, as an adult, when I wanted to speak Plautdietsch I had a block against it, a feeling of shame; I no longer spoke my mother tongue freely and fluently.

BIRTH PRACTICES

Since they deal with over sixty years of birth giving, these interviews describe many types of birthing practices and situations. The period discussed in these interviews (roughly 1920 to 1980) saw the end of home births (often attended by a doctor or midwife), the rise and dominance of modern hospital birthing techniques, and the gradual introduction of less-institutionalized birth practices, including the re-emergence of midwives in the 1970s.

Most members of my parents' generation were born at home, sometimes with a doctor for the first baby and a midwife thereafter. In fact, the same midwife attended the births of both of my parents — my great-grandmother,

Maria Heinrichs. (My father used to joke that his future grandmother-in-law spanked him when he was born.) Gradually, however, the hospital became the place where women went to give birth.

When my mother bore her first child in 1921, she was at her home in Halbstadt, Manitoba, attended by a doctor. Her next seven children were also born at home, often attended by Mrs. Wall, a midwife from the Halbstadt area. Fourteen years after the first birth, when they were expecting my arrival, my parents enrolled in a prepaid hospital insurance plan at Winnipeg's Concordia Hospital. As a result, when I was born in 1935 my mother had the luxury of a rest from household chores for ten days in the hospital before she boarded a train to return home with me in her arms.

What happened in the early part of the century to cause these women to turn to hospitals? The Mennonite midwives who served their communities around the turn of the century were no longer living by the time I began my interviews. Sara Kroeker describes how her mother and another woman responded to a call for volunteers in Steinbach to be trained in midwifery. Another practice, described by Margaret Sawatzky, involved "birthing homes," where one woman at a time went for her confinement and was attended by a doctor. In the 1930s and 1940s the first hospitals were built in small towns. Women went to them because they thought hospitals were cleaner and safer, and in some places the doctor's fee for a hospital birth was lower than for a home birth.

Beginning in the 1930s, hospital birth was seen as the modern choice. To women who became mothers during the next few decades, the decision of some of their daughters in the 1970s and 1980s to have home births seemed unsafe and even irresponsible, certainly a step backward. The women who had children between the 1940s and the 1970s were the most likely to have had anesthesia during childbirth, and in the course of these interviews they had the least to say about their birthing experiences. Some women experienced hospital births as profoundly alienating. Peggy Regehr and Robyn Epp found a lack of continuity of care and an absence of a personal relationship with care givers in a modern hospital.

A FINAL WORD

Just as I cannot now imagine life without my children, I cannot imagine life without having collected these birth stories. My horizons were widened; my capacity to listen compassionately without judgement was stretched. A strange phenomenon happened during these interviews: whether I knew the person or not, once I was seated across from her, listening to the story of her life, it was impossible not to feel empathy with her.

I feel fortunate to have heard the stories of the women represented here.

When I think of each of them, I can recall the season when we met, how I felt, and where I was in my continuing process of coming to terms with the material I was recording. I began the project with fear, but with time I realized the women's stories were central and that my role was only to facilitate. I learned that women may have essentially the same experience yet interpret it in very different ways. Karin Dirks, in my last interview, just before Christmas, added a joyous note with the German expression *Mutterwitz*, meaning the common sense passed on from one's mother, whose mother passed it on to her. *Mutterwitz* goes a long way.

I thank Heidi Harms, who initiated the process that led to the creation of this book. Her joy at discovering the many different voices confirmed my excitement about them. Without her, the stories would have languished longer before being in print.

Katherine Martens

Co-Editor's Note

THE CHALLENGE OF TRANSCRIBING IS to replicate on the page as faithfully as possible what has been recorded on tape. This is exacting work, even when one is trying to record only the actual words being spoken. Capturing on the page every pause, shift in tone, hesitation, and emotional nuance is quite impossible. Invariably I find it disappointing afterwards to read those neutral marks on the page — still hearing inwardly the rhythms and timbre of each woman's voice — and realizing that the general reader can never get the full effect.

Three of the interviews appearing here were conducted in German (Margaret Sawatzky, Helen Wedel, Gertrude Epp, all three immigrants from Ukraine in the 1920s), and two in Plautdietsch, or Mennonite Low German (Maria Reimer and Mrs. A, both born in Canada, also in the early 1900s). In these cases I translated into English as I went along, in effect doing a double translation, from one language and medium into another. An oral language like Plautdietsch, with its colourful expressions, is especially challenging. "Daut jeef noch een Jekaubel!" for example, loses something in spice, if not in meaning, in the translation to "There were quite some squabbles!" It is obvious in some of the interviews conducted in English that this was not the woman's first language, and a number of women seem unused to articulating their experiences, perhaps especially on the subject of giving birth.

As we edited the interviews for publication, we deleted repetitions and conversational quirks (such as "you know") as much as possible, and we occasionally rearranged sections for a better narrative flow. Fascinating as the stories woven in with the childbirth stories are, there simply wasn't room to include them all here, so many of these have been edited out. Throughout the editing process, our main concern was to preserve the distinctiveness of each woman's voice and to leave her story as intact as possible.

Although the work of transcribing is time-consuming and can be physically straining, those aspects were in this case quite eclipsed by the singular pleasure of listening to each conversation as it unfolded. Within minutes of beginning work on each interview, I felt drawn in, invited into an intimate conversation, spoken in accents and cadences as familiar to me as my own. I loved staying with each woman throughout the telling of her moving, heartbreaking, beautiful, individual story. I felt a link, listening to the older women especially, with my Mennonite heritage in a way I had not experienced before. Several times I became so overwhelmed with the richness and joy of it that I rewound part of the tape, telephoned a friend, and held the receiver to the tape recorder — once I even called my sister in Germany! — so that she could listen, too.

I gained a whole new appreciation for the interview as genre. Although the "conversation" is a staged one, with a very specific focus, there is a spontaneity in what is said, and especially in *how* it is said, that can't happen in other forms, such as the personal essay, for example. Much depends upon the interviewer to create the environment of mutual trust in which this staged-yet-spontaneous conversation can take place, and here my admiration and respect for Katherine's skills know no bounds.

I feel a huge gratitude toward Katherine for having initiated this very important project. Working with her has truly been a privilege and an inspiration.

Heidi Harms

In Her Own Voice

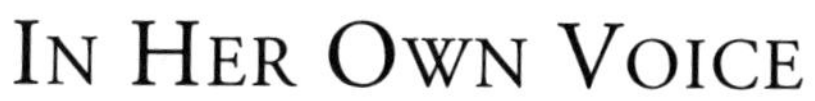

ANNA THIESSEN

Anna (Funk) Thiessen was born in Main Centre, Saskatchewan, in 1907. She and her husband, Cornelius, had ten children. She has lived in Plum Coulee and Winnipeg, and now lives in Steinbach, Manitoba.

Anna was my first interviewee, the big interview I had been working toward for months. I saw her in her comfortable apartment in Winnipeg with one of her daughters present. Anna spoke English and I thought I was well prepared for the interview, my question sheet within reach in case I needed it. We had set the stage during the pre-interview. What could go wrong except that everything I had learned in oral history workshops would fly out of my head at the last minute? Though I expected to hear her talk about both painful and joyful experiences, I think my mouth fell open when I heard her frank answer to my first question.

When you first found out you were pregnant, were you happy?
No. We have a family problem. My dad's grandparents married relatives. I knew it, and I didn't want to get married on account of that. Because my sisters had a couple of retarded children, and then I saw that and I didn't want to get married. But as it is, I did get married after all.

And were your children healthy then?
The first boy was very healthy. The second boy I noticed it right away that

there was retardation in there, and how I wished he could die rather than grow up, but he grew up to be fifty years. But we didn't have him at home all that time, we had to bring him away. We couldn't handle him. And then I was a person that got pregnant very quick, I got pregnant one after another. The first two were a year and three months apart, next one a year and five months, and I don't know how the fourth one was, I forget. Something like that, too.

Whom did you tell when you first got pregnant?
My husband. And I told him then right away, I said I was so scared for this and I didn't want it. He thought that I shouldn't be scared about it, it wouldn't always be like it. As it was just with the first children. And the last one. But that doctor told me that wasn't just that, it was because it was a very hard case . . . because he seemed to be all right sometimes, and next time he wasn't.

So the last child was a very difficult birth?
Yeah, it was a very difficult birth. That's the way it happened!

In what way was it difficult? Do you know the reason why?
Well, what I know — they did put me under a little bit — it came and then they pushed it back, it came and pushed it back in, until the doctor could get him. It took a long time.

Did you know anything about childbirth or pregnancy when you got married?
A little bit.

Did you know anything about family planning, birth control?
No. Not those years. I hardly think anybody knew about it.

Did your mother or your doctor or the midwife give you any advice ahead of time?
No. I didn't have a mother. My mother passed away before. And the midwife didn't tell me anything.

Did you see a midwife before you had the baby, or did she just come the day of the birth?
I went to a doctor before. I had a doctor for the last and the second last. They came to the house. And then the last child, the doctor said it was impossible at home. He took me to Winkler Hospital. And that's where I had him. That was Dr. B. from Winnipeg here; Dr. Wiebe was at the hospital,

but he was in parliament [Ed. note: Dr. Wiebe was an MLA at the time.] just exactly the days I had to go in. And Dr. R., he didn't know too much about it yet, he got mad and all kinds of things. I don't know why he was mad, I just couldn't do nothing with it. So — that's how it was.

Who delivered the other children then?
My husband's aunt, Mrs. Derksen. She was a midwife.

And none of them were unusually difficult?
Not to be born, no. I had very hard labour pains with some children, the first one and the fifth one. The twins were very easy, and — that's the way it went.

Did you continue working through your pregnancies?
Yes, we ran the farm, I worked all the time, and heavy too. After the birth, the tradition was at that time that we should stay in bed for ten days, but I never stayed in bed ten days. I was a strong person. Most of the time I felt very good, I worked very hard all through. I did my own washing, I did my water hauling, I worked on the field on account of that, it never bothered me.

Did anyone ever say to you, "Oh you're going to have a boy for sure because of the way you walk" or something like that?
Yes, but I didn't believe on it. [laughs] Never believed on it. I just thought to myself, nobody knows exact until it's born. I had a very good husband, he always looked very much after me, he was very careful. But you couldn't help this about this retarded. We couldn't do nothing about it except we could have, if we would have known what we know now we could have fixed it that I didn't have children any more.

What preparations did you make in your own house before the baby came?
I knew what I had to get, they told me. I had to get a big sheet of rubber sheeting, and then put an old blanket on top of that, and that's the way they were born, in bed at home.

What about your children? Did they stay home?
No, they were brought away. They were taken away to the neighbours'.

Were they told anything?
No. [laughs] That time it wasn't like it's now. Now they know it from the beginning on, that was not the case then. I never told the children anything

about it. My son always says now he didn't know, when he was thirteen years old he didn't even know. Because I never let on that I was pregnant or that I was going to have a baby or anything. See I was a person that didn't show, just the first one showed very much, but the other ones didn't. I was quite stout, and that's the way it went!

Do you remember something about each of the births of your children?
Well, the first one took an awful long time. It took from three o'clock in the afternoon till ten o'clock in the morning. And then my husband wanted to get a doctor, but then those old wives said, "No, don't get a doctor, it's not necessary." And they wouldn't let him get a doctor. And the second one came easy, it didn't take long. And the third one wasn't too heavy either. Fourth one was, well it started up one time and went away and after a week it started up again and then he came. And then we didn't have nobody there, nobody got ready that time. My husband and his sister did it, his sister was living with us. And then after that one — who was it now — oh, Annie was very hard. My daughter. That was a very long case too. She was born in July, and we called the doctor yet, but he was with another woman, so he couldn't come right away, and when he came she was born already. That midwife, she knew what to do, she did all she could. She said just that we had to get a doctor, so we did. And then the next ones were the twins, and they were so easy, I just thought I was going into diarrhea when I got them! [laughs] got the twins. And one came an hour and a half later than the other.

Did you know ahead of time that you were going to have twins?
Yes. That I knew. I always said, that does not give me rest, there must be two. I never got rest. Kept on moving all the time. And nobody told me that it would be twins, but I knew by myself it must be twins. And then when they were born I had everything ready, like for blue and pink, and they thought, how did you know that you were going to have twins? Well, I said, I wasn't sure, but I was thinking of it. Oh how I wished then that they were the last ones! After the twins I had about three yet. I had ten children all together. I don't think I ever lost one. Except the last one, before my operation. I was so sick and the doctor said that I had a growth and they would have to take it out, and then they found another baby there. That was quite an ordeal there.

So it was stillborn.
Well — I don't know for sure if it was stillborn, I just heard the doctor say to the other doctor if he would have known he would have waited yet. It

would have had to die anyways because it could not be born like that, with the growth inside. Quite a big tumour. And I thought that was the last one, it was the last one. He fixed me up then right away.

When you were at home for your births, were you able to move around or did you stay strictly in bed?
No, I moved around as long as I could. The midwives always told me it was better for me. And I did what they told me. They said I should move around as much as I could and as long as I could. When I had one boy I took so terrible long I couldn't stay up, I had to lie down, because I was going to faint all the time. Finally he was born, six o'clock in the evening.

Did you ever have help in your house after a child came?
Yes, I had — oh I think I had about three or four maids.

And then later of course the children got old enough to help.
Yes. But there was milking to do and everything, and I never waited very long until I went back to work. I was a person, I worked very quick, it never bothered me, work, but I always told my husband that if I would have known it I sure would not have gotten married. But he always tried to tell me, oh that won't bother us. But as it is, that's the way it was.

So other than the retardation, were there other sicknesses, childhood illnesses that gave you a lot of concern?
No, my family was very healthy. Well, of course the measles and chicken pox and that yeah, but I don't believe that is a sickness, it comes too naturally to children. But otherwise they were healthy. Except the second one, he was never healthy.

Did you tell your son about your family history?
Oh yes. [laughs] I told him this all, I said, "Think of it, what's in our family, in case you should have children like that, how heavy that is to go through." I was so scared when I found out I was pregnant, this is going to be it again, and like Dr. M. told my friend, they had the harelip in their family, and he says, "As long as you think it could be harelip, you will have it. Get off of it." I couldn't, I tried to get rid of that thinking it could be a retarded one again, it seemed I couldn't.

You were saying that you'll never forget the first birth, it was a very unusual experience. Can you say some more about that one?
That afternoon I told my husband — his parents had visitors — I said, "I

hope they don't stay overnight, it feels like if I'm going to go into labour." And he said, "Oh no, let's hope it won't." And sure enough it did. And then my mother-in-law would not let me stay upstairs, like we had the room upstairs. She would not let me stay upstairs, I had to come down, because she was a heavy, sickly woman, and she didn't want to run upstairs always. So I got more in pain, I walked around upstairs, I didn't say nothing. I tried to hold my mouth, I wasn't going to holler out loud. All of a sudden, she must have noticed it, and I called down to see what she would say and I asked her what was wrong with me, whether it was the labour pains or not, and she said yes, it must be. I said, "What are you going to do with the visitors?" She said, "Just change them for upstairs, and you come down." She had told me that much what I had to get ready, so I got that sheet of rubber ready and the blanket and everything I had ready. And she sat down, because she said she couldn't sleep anyway, she was so worried about me. And then I said to my husband, I said, "It's coming on stronger and stronger, what am I going to do with those visitors upstairs? I can't take that." That was the middle of the night, that was in January, and an awful big snowstorm, we couldn't do much, except he could have gotten the doctor, with horses and sleigh, because it was in the country village, and it was too hard to walk for a doctor. He wasn't young any more. So then, we'll see. We'll see, that's what always came, the words. Just wait. Give it time, another hour. I told that midwife, I says, "You think that I can scream another hour? I can't, then I wish I'd die." My husband says, "Oh no, I don't want you to!" But it went on further and further, and then in the morning when those people got up, that man said, "I never heard a thing like that in my life! We never went through such a thing as this." And they left for my mother-in-law's brother, he lived two houses off, that's where they went then. He said, "Boy, such a thing I've never heard. Such a terrible thing." I have a loud voice as it is, so I must have been terrible. But finally, at ten o'clock in the morning, just when the clock stroked ten, he came. I always tease him with that.

Was that the one you had the dream about ahead of time?
Yeah. That was when I had the dream that the stovepipes were so hard to come through, something wanted to come through there, I didn't know what, but it was so hard, and it couldn't get through and couldn't get through, and finally he got through. And then after I was well, I told my husband what I had dreamt that night. And he says, that sure was tough!

You were only seventeen.
Yes.

You mentioned that they had certain practices that they did with babies. What were they?
Well, I don't know, there wasn't much, they just rolled them in very tightly and put a hot water bottle around them and said it should be good and warm.

Did you worry about screaming at home, or did it not bother you?
No. Didn't bother me one bit, I didn't care. If it helped me anything I screamed. 'Course you couldn't be quiet. With nothing to take or nothing to do, anything, no needle or anything, it was just terrible. I sometimes wonder how I ever did it, with ten children, did all the work and milking and everything. But I did it. 'Course I was a very strong woman. I still am strong, but I can't walk.

Margaret Sawatzky

Margaret (Klassen) Sawatzky was born in southern Russia in 1909. She lived in Gnadenthal in southern Manitoba for many years and now lives in Winnipeg. She married in 1933, and she and her husband, Bernhard, have eleven children.

I met with Mrs. Sawatzky in snowy February, once to get acquainted with her and again the following week for the recording. The fact that she knew my parents inspired her to have confidence in me. Margaret Sawatzky spoke High German, which was a challenge to me. I had learned German reasonably well in school, in church, and during sojourns in Germany, but I had to face my fear of making a mistake. At first I was inhibited and stumbled over die, der, *and* das. *Both of us were nervous for different reasons, but as the interview progressed we relaxed. The visit with her, as well as with other older women, even women who in the end did not give me an interview, were of immense importance to me. Their homespun wisdom, their outlook on life which reminded me of my mother, together with their willingness to talk frankly to me, a stranger, are gifts.*

[Translated from German]

Mrs. Sawatzky, when you learned that you were pregnant, how did you feel? Well, my feelings were quite varied. Actually I had more trouble with pregnancy than with childbirth. I was sick a lot during my pregnancies.

And when I noticed that I was pregnant — I usually noticed in my second month — my husband always knew right away too, of course, but I would tell my mother and my sisters.

What did you know about childbirth at the time you got married?
Well, actually I knew almost nothing about it. I was the third youngest in the family and my sisters all had children, all had families, but I didn't really have any idea what was involved.

And birth control, did you know anything about that?
No, we didn't have anything like that, we used no birth control at that time.

What were your expectations about pregnancy, about becoming a mother?
Well, we looked forward to our babies. The first one, we were very happy about it, and later, too. Actually God has arranged things in such a way that you love the little children, once they are growing in your body! And even if things seemed difficult at times, I never wished that it should be born dead, or that it not be born at all; we looked forward to the children.

When you were pregnant, could you move about like usual?
Yes, I worked as much as I could. I milked cows, sometimes up to the last morning, I would be milking the cow in the morning and I would say to my husband, today is the day. I could feel it already. But the cow finished being milked despite that, and everything got done until you knew, now is the time.

I guess the first child was a little easier, the pregnancy, because there were no other children yet.
I had a midwife, I wanted her to attend the birth, but for the first two she wouldn't do it, it was her opinion that I would want to have an anesthetic. And she wasn't able to administer it. So the doctor had to come from Winkler, Dr. Wiebe, he came out just for the birth.

And did you receive anesthesia?
They gave me chloroform. With the first baby, my husband was actually anesthetized more quickly than I was, he was supposed to hold the lamp, it was a kerosene lamp, and all of a sudden he started to sway, so he had to be taken out of the room. [laughs] And the child was born in the near darkness, but it was born, after a while.

Did you have any fears?
Well, yes, it did seem difficult. But we had faith in God, and that helped us through many things.

You said before that your husband was present during the births of your children.
Yes. My husband was always present, I almost ripped his arms off! That was what I held onto!

And did that help?
Yes. Yes, that helped. And that was a big part of it, that we experienced it together.

I think that's lovely. Who else was there?
When the midwife didn't come, my mother helped too. She would be there for the first few days and look after the baby. My husband would look after me. And the midwife had instructed me to stay in bed for one week after. The doctor didn't really say much about how long one should stay in bed. But because I had had stitches, I couldn't get up any sooner. And I have to say one more thing: when the midwife looked after me, she prayed the whole time, and once the baby was born, she knelt down beside the bed and thanked God for being with us and that the baby had come into the world, and that child and mother were alive. And that gave strength. She was an educated midwife, she had studied in Russia, she was a very devout woman. Her name was Mrs. Janzen from Gnadenthal. We lived in the village of Gnadenthal at that time.

Were your children present as well?
Once there were children they would be brought to other family members when a new baby was about to be born. And sometimes I needed some help afterwards, when I was bedridden, and that would usually be my nieces from Blumenort. They helped out in a very loving way. And that created a bond between us so that even now, whenever they have the chance, they call me or come over, and we stay in touch with each other. And I think that had a lot to do with it, we became friends at that time. We carried it all more or less together. And when the baby was going to be born at home we would get a little anxious every evening, we wouldn't know of course exactly when it was going to happen, but the house would always have to be put in order. Before we went to bed everything had to be tidied, the floor wiped; clothing for the baby would have been prepared ahead of time, so that one could go to bed in peace, even if the stork should suddenly arrive. [laughs] Actually we didn't believe in the stork, but that was an old saying.

What do you remember about an individual birth, or several, anything in particular?

Well, there were all kinds of things. I had twins, and I had already been in the hospital for a few days, but then it stopped, so I came home again for Sunday, we had company on Sunday, and then a few days later it started again. So we drove off to Altona to the hospital. At first we had no hospital, not in Altona or in Winkler. There were houses where pregnant women could go and have their babies. And when I came, there was a hospital in Altona, it was a private home that had been renovated, and on the second story was the delivery room, and so we had to go up the stairs. But that morning when we had just set out, my pains stopped again, and I said to my husband, "It's going to be for nothing again." He stopped the car, and we stayed there and watched the sun rise in the east. And we sat and chatted about this and that, and suddenly the cramps started again. And I said, "Now let's go!" So we drove very fast, but it was not too fast! When we got there the nurse was glad to see it was as far along as it was, and so I gave birth to the first baby, and twenty minutes later the second. And the nurses were very good. It was Dr. Toni from Altona who looked after me.

We had to stay in the hospital for such a long time. Usually for ten days, but I was in for up to twelve days. And so we got to know our fellow patients very well. There were usually four women in a room, we had a lot of fun. Once the birth is over, you're not sick, maybe a bit weak, but we were in bed. So we had good conversations there, and the nurses would come and cheer us up. Quite often they would come in and say, "Oh, we've brought you such nice pillowcases, now you're going to feel great!" And it did cheer us up.

Who made the decisions about how long you stayed in bed after the birth, the doctor?

Yes, mostly the doctor. In the hospital, Dr. Toni would always say, if the tenth day was a Sunday, and you really wanted to go home, he would say, "Wait until the sun comes up, and then you can go." But it had to be ten days. And after the twins were born, he said, no, I would have to stay twelve days. And they would also pass.

Did the doctor or the midwife always come on time?

Yes, in our case they usually had to wait a bit yet. When Dr. Wiebe came, he would even help heat up the brick stove. The first child was born in April, that was a very hot day, but another one was born in September, and the weather was cold and rainy. And he said, "It's much too cold!" We used a brick stove for heating, and he found that very interesting. He saw I wasn't quite ready yet, so he sat by the brick stove and kept heating it.

So even when you were attended by a doctor, it was sometimes at home, not necessarily in the hospital.
Yes. Yes. With the first two the doctor came to me. And Dr. Wiebe would — once the baby was born, it would need a bath, right? but he would rub baby oil on it, all over the baby's body, and then he wiped it off and rolled the baby in a blanket, and then it was clean! [laughs] Who will have dressed the baby properly—maybe my husband, I don't know, I've forgotten; I would still be preoccupied with myself!

Did you ever scream?
I can't say if I screamed, but I certainly groaned loudly. [laughter]

When you were in the hospital, did you find that easier or more difficult?
Well, I'm not really sure. At first I always thought that would be very cumbersome, going to the hospital once labour had begun. But later we got used to that, too; we gladly went to the hospital, it was good, it was very good. Birth at home didn't really work any more, the family was bigger, you couldn't take six, seven children out at night.

How long did the doctor usually stay?
Usually until everything was over, the afterbirth and everything had been looked after, then he'd leave.

And the midwife?
The midwife would come over every morning for a whole week, she would come and bathe the baby and look after me, my husband would have to go pick her up with the buggy, she lived in the same village.

Did you breast-feed your children?
Yes, I breast-fed the first few, about up to one year. But later on the milk didn't come in, so they had to have bottles, and later with Pablum and so on.

Earlier we talked about convalescent homes. Could you tell me what that means?
Yes, in those days not every small town had a hospital, and so homes were opened up where women could go to deliver their babies. In Gretna there were Helen and Sarah Heinrichs, they had a home, and women would go there if it wasn't possible for them to stay at home for the birth. My own

sister was there several times, and she has very good memories about it. I visited her there, and I think these homes did very good work. In Altona there were the Nickel sisters, they also took in women who were about to give birth, I have also visited people there. And they had their place. When the hospitals were built, of course they weren't as big as they are now, in Winkler it had four rooms, in Altona a private home was set up as a hospital, and later fine hospitals were built. But in those days the convalescent homes did their work, too, their duty. I think they did very good work.

When your children were a bit older, would they notice when you were pregnant?
They say actually that they never noticed anything different about me, they always thought I couldn't walk very well, they had to help more, but that a little baby was coming, that was something they were not told ahead of time. But they were always happy. I remember especially when the eleventh baby was born, when my husband returned from the hospital and told them a little baby sister had arrived in the hospital, they tell me how they jumped about for joy. And that's how they would come to meet me in the car, when I returned with the little baby, and they loved it very much, and they still love her, even though she's over thirty by now.

Are you happy to be a mother?
Oh yes. I can't imagine my life without my children. And I don't have one too many! Especially now that I'm a widow, I need all of them. Once one child can come and help, another time someone else, so they all get a turn. And earlier, too, when they were still small, not one was too many. After they were all in bed, my husband and I would often go with the lamp and look at the children while they slept, tuck them under the covers again, and were happy.

And are you a grandmother yet?
Yes, I'm a grandmother. And I'm also a great-grandmother, I already have two great-grandchildren, and one on the way. You love the grandchildren I think just the same as you loved your children. And what makes me happy is that they also like me.

Helen Wedel

Helen (Klassen) Wedel was born in Omsk, Russia, in 1906 and lived in Siberia before she immigrated to Manitoba in the twenties. She and her husband, Jacob, had five children.

When I visited Helen Wedel in her Winnipeg apartment, she was in the process of writing her memoirs for her children and grandchildren, so our interview seemed almost effortless to me. She talked without prompting and I enjoyed the stories. As someone whose cookie jar is often empty, I have an uncanny memory for all the homes where I was offered tea and cookies. Helen was expecting her grandchild to come for lunch. I was reminded of a visit to my grandmother when I was little. The memory of sitting at her table for an hour to listen spellbound to her life story is imprinted on my mind as an image of the link between the generations. Not included here, but in the full taped version of Helen's interview, is her account of her parents' narrow escape from Russia. Had she lived in less troubled times, Helen would have studied medicine.

[Translated from German]

Why did you come to Canada earlier than your parents did?
Yes, there was a reason for that. I already had a boyfriend. We were not officially engaged, but we had promised each other that we wanted to marry some day. We felt we were too young yet, though. And so we decided, since

his parents were going, and he didn't want me to stay there, that we would come here and maybe take jobs for two years or so, pay our travel loans, and then get married. Which is what we did. We got married after two years, had paid our travel loans, and settled on a farm near Wawanesa, about thirty miles from Brandon. We had lived there for a whole year when my parents came. They arrived in September of 1929. I was expecting my first child shortly. The other siblings already had families, they didn't have room on the farm. We had room, and so we took in my parents.

When you first realized that you were pregnant, how did you feel?
Oh, I was happy, in one way, knowing that I was going to have a child. But I was so inexperienced. I had no difficulties with pregnancy, but I had trouble with my stomach, I had to watch very carefully what I ate. I often thought, I wonder what this child is going to look like, it won't look healthy. But he was a very beautiful round boy, the first one. That was my first birth, we were living on the farm, and we were poor, because we had to see that we paid off the farm, so we decided that I would stay at home.

We had a doctor four miles away in Wawanesa. I went to see him a few times while I was pregnant. He said everything was in order, he would come to our house, and everything should be just fine. And then my parents arrived that fall, in September, and at the end of October my son was born. My parents came and lived with us, so I had my mother there, that was very nice. She told me a lot of things that I should do, and prepared everything for the birth. Because it was taking place at home, I had to be in bed. She sewed together layers of paper and old sheets that we could discard after.

I had actually thought it would be on the third of November, but it happened a bit earlier. I made a joke the night before. I went outside, there was no snow yet, it was the 30th of October, and I said to my husband, "Well, who knows, tomorrow is Hallowe'en, maybe our boy will come tomorrow and shout 'Hallowe'en!'" [laughs] Well, we laughed about that, didn't think it would happen, but really, the next morning when I woke up I could feel the labour pains already. It was early, five o'clock, and they were spaced evenly already, with some time in between, but by breakfast time they were not quite as frequent. After breakfast my husband said, "I'll go and get the doctor anyway." It had started to snow, and was snowing quite heavily by then. So he went to get the doctor, and unfortunately the regular doctor was not home. He was a young man, and he had just got married and hadn't returned from his honeymoon yet. Well, what now? So they had told him, "Go there and there, there's an old doctor there, he's retired, but maybe he'll come with you, he's done a lot of this kind of work." The old doctor was quite reluctant, didn't really want to do it, but let himself be talked into it and came with him. They went to the young doctor's office and picked up some equipment. I was very glad.

The labour pains had decreased. They got home between ten and eleven in the morning. The doctor sat down beside my bed and asked me all kinds of questions, he was very interested in the fact that we had come from Russia, so we talked a lot. By lunchtime the pains had got so mild that he said, "I'm going to go home and come back in the afternoon, let me know if the pains get more severe." And so that's what he did, he drove home, but the weather had turned stormy, the wind had picked up and the snow was falling more heavily. So he came again in the afternoon, we telephoned him, my husband called from the neighbours' house. The pains were getting more and more intense, and finally he said, "Yes, it's going to be soon now." So he stayed there until he was born, at five o'clock that afternoon. It was storming quite badly by then, and the doctor was restless to get home. So he just did what was absolutely necessary, he attended to me, the afterbirth was taken care of, he gave my mother some instructions about the immediate care, and then he drove home.

Well, I was very happy that it was all over, and I was very grateful to God. Everything was normal. He was a nice, beautiful, big boy of nine and a half pounds, which we hadn't counted on, nice and round and healthy. I stayed in bed for a few days, and the nice thing about being at home, which I found out later — I had four more children, all of them in the hospital in Winnipeg, and they wouldn't let us get out of bed! We had to stay in bed for nine days. And that made me sick. When I was at home, I could get up on the second day, after a few days I started walking around, and everything was fine. There were no complications. Of course it would have been different if there had been complications. But everything went very well. And I would often say to the nurses here in Winnipeg, "Let me get up! Nothing will happen to me, I've tried it once before!" No, those were their rules, and they had to be followed. So we were only allowed to get up for the first time after nine days, and then go home on the tenth day.

Did you have the feeling that you had enough information about pregnancy and childbirth?

Yes, I did, I had the feeling that I knew enough. Although I didn't know everything! But I don't know, I suppose I've always been quite self-assured. Also I had read a lot about it, I knew the main things about it, and I also tried to do all the right things during my pregnancy, and I felt quite confident that everything would go well. The doctor had said that everything was normal, and so I had no worries. I'm not the type of person who worries a lot, I am not easily worried, I take life from "the opposite side." [laughs]

Did you know anything about birth control?
No. Oh no, we didn't have that then.

But you did not have many children.
No, but I did know this: in the Bible we have birth control. And one day my granddaughter wanted to know, so I told her, "You know, we didn't have any birth control except for the Biblical ones. God already told Israel, the women have their times, and for such and such a time men are not to come to the women. And that's what that is about. If you follow that, you will not become pregnant, after."

And did you breast-feed?
Yes, I breast-fed them all for just over a year. I had lots of milk. — But I also had two miscarriages, after the oldest. Once I was just two months pregnant, I lifted something that was too heavy and lost the baby, and once I was three months pregnant. By then we were living here in Winnipeg. The doctor told me to be very careful the next time. And so with my daughter, that was six years later, I had to be very careful.

You've said that you are very interested in nutrition and health. Did you read about diet during pregnancy?
Oh yes! I had several books from Germany that I had brought with me from Russia, and read them: lots of milk, for calcium — and I still didn't drink enough milk, the way it was on the farm, the cows were dry, and you couldn't just buy it like that, so that my teeth suffered from that. But the child was strong and healthy. After the first child I didn't lose any teeth, but with the other children I lost several teeth after each birth. But since the youngest was born, forty-three years ago, I haven't lost any teeth.

So you just continued working as usual through your pregnancy?
Yes, I worked hard! We had a huge garden on the farm, and we helped outside as much as possible, my sisters-in-law and I, we milked the cows, looked after the chickens, and did everything. And it didn't hurt me at all. I was used to the work. But we only stayed on the farm for three years. Right in the first year, while my husband was lifting up an old granary, levering it up, he slipped and a big beam fell against his side and damaged his kidney. So he had a lot of infections in those years, and because the field work was still done with horses in those days, the vibrations were so bad that he was

always getting kidney infections. And finally the doctor told him, "If you want to live, you'll have to leave the farm." He had already been a teacher for two years in Russia as a young man, and he was much more interested in teaching than in farming. I asked him before we got married, "Wouldn't you rather study here and become a teacher?" "No," he said, "I want to farm." He had worked for some English farmers, farming was going well in those years, and they had said, "Stay on the farm, that way you're your own boss. If you become a teacher you'll always be bossed around by trustees and others. And that's no good." So he didn't want to, but his real interest lay in school. Well, I told him later, the dear Lord had known where he belonged. So finally after three years we left the farm. How we managed to get through without any debts was like a miracle of God. That was already the Depression, everyone was astounded that we would leave the farm with nothing. A little bit of cash, but with empty hands, and despite that we always managed.

Were there any kinds of popular sayings or beliefs, like predicting that you would have a boy or a girl?
Oh, we had a joke, maybe I should tell it now. My brother-in-law, the one we lived with, had bought a small hatching machine for hatching baby chicks on the farm. And someone had told him that he could tell by the eggs whether they would produce a rooster or a hen. It was a small thing, about the size of a fifty-cent piece, round, tied to a string; he was to hold this over the egg, and if it was going to be a rooster — now I'm not sure, did it turn in circles then or did it go back and forth, but in one case it went one way and in another the other way. And that's how he could test the eggs. And he got mostly baby hens, not roosters. And then one day, I was quite far along in my pregnancy, probably in my seventh month or so, and his wife was just in the beginning, it was also her first, they were talking about this business of testing the eggs. "Oh," my husband says suddenly, "we should test our wives! Maybe that'll show too!" Well, we all laughed about it and didn't believe it at all. "No way," I said, "that's just silliness." But they insisted, so we let ourselves be persuaded, and each man tested his wife. And sure enough, mine showed that I would have a boy and hers that she would have a girl, and that's how it was.

Really?! [laughter]
Yes! They held it over our bodies, just the way they had held it over the eggs, and it showed! So I counted on having a boy. — But apart from that, I don't know. Yes, that was fun.

During labour, did you move around or were you in bed?
I was in bed and had to lie on my side. That didn't please me at all, but this

was an old English doctor, and he had brought this method with him from England, and he said it had to be done this way and it was easier for the woman. But I didn't believe him. My back almost broke in half.

And the other births?

They were all here in Winnipeg, in the Concordia Hospital, all four. For the first daughter I had Dr. Klassen, he was a very good women's doctor, we loved him very much, it was a pity he had to die so young. And that birth was normal. There was some fun with that one, too. She was supposed to be born in May, but I actually thought it would be a few days later. She was born on May 29. I never got very big, it wasn't obvious that I was as far along as I was. We were with our first school, my husband had a position by now, he had finished his studies and had gotten his first school, and we lived on the schoolyard there. And one day some people from Steinbach came over, they had heard that we were interested in buying a car, and they were car dealers. And it was just recess time. So I invited them in, they sat down, my husband came in and they started talking, and my husband said, "Yes, I can't be without a car, I'll need it any time." "Why?" the man asked. "Well, I'll have to go to Winnipeg any time with my wife, she's expecting a baby." Both of them looked at me and the woman said, "No, that can't be." She had thought, while following me into the house, she almost looks as if she might be pregnant. But that I was almost full term? No, that was impossible. "Yes," I said, "it's true. I expect it to be this week, or next week at the latest."

So they went to Winnipeg and returned in the evening and said there was a car in Winnipeg, if we were interested, they could take us there to look at it. So my husband said to me, "Take all your things with you and you can stay there already." My father and my sisters were living in Kildonan [a part of Winnipeg]. The woman says to me on the way, "If it's really true that you're about to have a baby, please let me know. I've never seen anything like this, for a woman to be showing so little this close to the birth." That was Wednesday, and on Thursday she was born. Right the next day. I took the taxi to Kildonan, and the next day I had to go to the hospital. My husband was still in school with the oldest boy, they would be coming in Friday after four.

Dr. Klassen lived across the street from the Concordia Hospital. So they come in Friday after four, and my husband sees Dr. Klassen out in the garden. He goes over and Dr. Klassen shakes his hand and says, "Congratulations on your daughter!" My husband gives him a baffled look and says, "What are you talking about?" "Well!" he says, "don't you know yet? You have a big daughter!" "Oh, you're joking!" "No," says the doctor, "She's right here in the Concordia!" "Oh!" says my husband, "I just wanted to tell you that my wife is here and is waiting!" [laughs] And so he came into the hospital all excited. — Yes, a big girl, nine pounds. The oldest was nine and a half. All my babies were big, except for the second daughter, she was eight pounds. The third daughter was also nine and a half pounds, and the youngest boy was almost ten.

When he was born here in the hospital, that's another story. We were at the school in Osborne at the time. I had been splitting wood. We had guests and there was no wood; we still used wood-burning stoves, and I wanted to make *Faspa* (afternoon lunch). Usually my husband kept the box full of firewood, but now there was none. So I quickly into the cellar and start splitting wood. And it was so hard, I almost couldn't do it, but I managed. This was about two weeks before the baby was due. Right away on Monday my labour pains started. So my husband says, "We'll take you in." "No," I said. With my other daughter I had waited for two weeks in Winnipeg, because I had had a fall and had dislocated it, and she was born two weeks later than her due date. Well, he was a little anxious, he came in at every recess. I was working as hard as I could, cleaning and baking *Zwieback* (rolls) and getting everything ready, because we had made arrangements to have a girl come in from La Salle, but she was only supposed to come in two weeks! So there wouldn't be anybody, and there were already four children. "Oh," says my husband, "it will all work out. I'll take you in or I'll put you on the train." We lived very near the station, and the train left at noon. No, I didn't want that. So we waited until after four, and then my husband said, "I'll go over to the neighbours', the Rempels, and see if Liese is available just in case we have to leave suddenly." So he took the bicycle over there.

While he was gone, I prayed, "Dear God, if this is really the time, please send me a labour pain that will make me know for sure." And sure enough, I had such a strong pain that I had to lie down. So now I knew. I quickly washed and changed my clothes, and our second daughter, who always noticed everything, she was very lively, came in and said, "Mama, what are you doing?" I said, "I want to go to the hospital and get the baby." I had been telling them for a while that we would be getting a new baby. "I want to come too!" "No, child, you cannot come with me, I'm going to have to stay there for awhile, and you can't come with me." She was only five years old, I hadn't explained it to her yet. I had told the oldest ones, but not her. So I said, "I'll bring home a beautiful boy." I had the feeling it was going to be another boy; I'd had three girls in a row and wanted to have a boy. Well, she cried a bit, but the others were staying home too, the oldest one was thirteen by now, and I told her, "Liese Rempel will come over, Papa has gone to ask her, she'll come here for night." Well, it was all settled, I finished changing my clothes, gave the children fresh buns and milk. Then my husband came in and saw everything, and said, "Na?" and I said, "Well, let's go."

It had been raining for several days, the ruts in the road were deep, and we had eighteen miles to go before the highway. There was gravel, but not much. The first few miles were all right, but then the ruts got deeper, and each time there was such a bump. My pains got so strong at one point, I said, "I'm not sure I can hold on." "Please try!" he said. At first I had planned on lying down in the back of the car, but then I remembered something my sister-in-law had once told me: "If you're that close to delivery, don't lie down in the car. Stay upright, and you can hold onto it a bit longer." And I knew that if I were to lie down, it would have been born in the car. — Well, we hadn't gone very far yet, and it got quite bad, the urge to push started. Usually I had only one or two pushes and then the baby was there. My husband just couldn't see his way through, and drove as hard as he could. When we finally got to Winnipeg — I had managed to suppress one of the push urges, I pressed down hard on the seat and prayed — we got into the city, and when we got to the parliament building there was suddenly a police officer there, there were traffic lights, but we were not stopping anywhere, we just went right through. The policeman was right behind us on his big motorcycle, and followed us all the way to the Concordia, and my husband stopped and ran in. The policeman just looked inside the car and asked no questions.

And then when we stopped it let up a bit, I had suppressed it so hard. Two nurses came running out to the car to help me, and I said, "Oh, just now the pains are gone, I can walk in by myself." They each took an arm and helped me along, but just at that moment the pain was gone completely. They took me into the hospital, and had a long discussion about which room they would put me in, and I said, "Just put me in the birthing room, that's where I want to go. With the next push the baby is going to be there." Well, they didn't want to believe me because I wasn't having any pain at the moment. I told them, "I've been suppressing it, if I hadn't it would have already happened." They finally believed me and took me to the birthing room. The head nurse went to phone the doctor right away; he was out of town and unavailable, so she phoned another one, and nothing was ready! The nurses were a bit flustered, they were just changing shifts. They brought me in, and I quickly undressed, and suddenly, I was still wearing my corset and my stockings, and I could feel, here it comes! So I up on the table, and just then a practical nurse comes running in from the hall. "The baby's coming!" And the head nurse tells her — she's standing in the hallway — "Push it back!" She grabbed a piece of cotton wool and pushed it back. And the pains stopped instantly. But that should not have happened! And then it took just minutes. My husband had heard this, he heard me screaming and that the baby was coming, and then everything was quiet. So he was alarmed by this, and ran across the street to the nurses' home, there was an old nurse named Johanna who lived there. He just asked, "Where is Sister Johanna?" and he brought her in, and just as she was entering, the baby started coming for the second time, and again the head nurse told the practical nurse, "Push it back." She was just getting her cotton wool again when the door opened and Johanna came in. She grabbed the practical nurse by the arm and yanked her away and said, "No more pushing back here!" And as she was speaking, the baby was there. That's how quickly it happened. That nurse, as well as the head nurse, was laid off later. That was very dangerous, they said. — He was a big boy, almost ten pounds. But that was an experience I will never forget!

It was early evening, between seven and eight o'clock, when he was born, and that night I got no sleep at all. I was so agitated, they tried giving me sleeping pills, but they didn't help at all, I couldn't sleep at all. And the doctor never came, Johanna took the baby, and everything was fine. It was normal, and she waited until the afterbirth had come out, and she said that everything was fine, she brought me to my bed, and the next morning at ten o'clock Dr. Oelkers came by. "Well!" he said, "you surprised us!" "Yes," I said, "and me too!" [laughs]

The child wanted to be born!
Yes, and he was hungry all the time, because he was so big. At that time they had this wagon that they put all the babies on to roll them into the rooms, and they always put him first, at the front. The nurses would say, "Here comes the big policeman, he's so hungry already!" Yes, that was quite an experience.

Did you moan and scream?
Yes, I screamed. But these days they say it's not necessary, you don't have to scream. For example, my daughter says they practise beforehand and try it, and they do not need to scream. I say I don't know, I did it without wanting to, it happened all by itself. The push urges were so strong, and I had to scream. My mother did too. And I've read about that in the Bible, too, women screaming in childbirth. So I suppose it's normal. Whenever the push urges came on, I would scream, loudly. It gave me some relief.

Maybe it can be harmful not to scream, if one wants to.
Yes, I think so. My daughter has had very quick births, just a few labour pains, she almost doesn't make it to the hospital in time, and then the baby is there. She doesn't have long labours like I did — well, with my youngest

one the labour wasn't as long, but when she was born, that was the most difficult birth, and she was the smallest one. But I had such terrible labour pains, a whole day and a whole night, I was so exhausted, I had hardly any strength left.

Are you happy to be a mother? Can you imagine your life without your children? No, I can't imagine my life without my children, and I have always been very happy with my children. I always looked forward to them, and also to my grandchildren and great grandchildren. I love children very much. And I am very glad to have had my own children. I have often felt sorry for people who had no children.

Sara Kroeker

Sara (Reimer) Kroeker was born in Steinbach, Manitoba, in 1905 and lived there all her life. She and her husband, Peter, had nine children. I saw Sara and Maria Reimer, her good friend, on the same days. They were both wise women for me, and when I'm in despair the image of these two women gives me hope.

By this time I was beginning to realize that the more questions I asked and the more detailed the notes I made in the pre-interview, the better and more rounded out the recorded interview would be. Earlier I mistakenly thought the actual interview might be anticlimactic if we covered too much ground in the pre-interview. Memory has a way of drifting and coming back in layers, and the week between the two sessions often helped the process.

Sara spoke English with an overlay of "Mennonite" constructions — for example, "Oh, and you're here yet even if Sara felt it all night already?" which translates into "You're here in spite of the fact that Sara had labour pains all night?"

Much of Sara's interview includes stories of her mother, Aganetha Reimer, a midwife for many years in the Steinbach area.

My mother, Aganetha Barkman, was the daughter of Jakob Barkman, she was born in 1863 in Rückenau, southern Russia. My mother grew up as a healthy and an active child, and when she was about nine or ten years old, she saw how her brothers were swimming in the Dnieper River there, and she was really interested in this, and asked her brother to show her how to swim too, and he said, "OK, Neet, just come into the water, and I'll teach you how to swim." And she went in, he took her into the deep, and then he said, "Neet, nü schwam, oda dü fesipst!" ("Sink or swim, Nettie!"). Well, of course, she wouldn't drown there, she just struggled out of the deep and learned how to swim!

My mother grew up, and there happened to be a widower in the village by the name of John R. Reimer. And of course, they would go and help this widower, he had four little girls from three to seven years of age. They would help him, whatever they could do for him, and girls would have to go and clean up there and do some washing and baking for him, and also my mother. And eventually Mr. Reimer, he kind of liked this girl, and eventually he married her. Then she had these four little girls to take care of, and also there was a lot of work to do outside, she really liked to work outside, too, help her husband, in whatever way she could.

And eventually she had her own family; and when she had five children, then the question came up in the whole group of Steinbach that they really needed a midwife very badly. They didn't have doctors around, and they had heard of a lady in Minnesota, a Mrs. Neufeld, who was really called a doctor with all her home remedies and experience, and then the congregation decided that they would let this Mrs. Neufeld come out to Steinbach. And now was the thing, would there be a volunteer to learn for this thing as a midwife. And my mother wanted to, she would do that. So my mother and a certain Mrs. Peter Toews from Greenland also came for these lessons, and they took lessons around three weeks, many home remedies were written down.

Do you have any of these home remedies yet, do you have copies of them?
Yeah, she copied them in the same book where she afterwards copied all the births that she delivered.

How many were there?
Well, she delivered around a good 600 babies that she registered. Afterwards, there were a few, mostly her grandchildren, she hadn't registered them. She had many experiences as a midwife. Sometimes she would go out to the surrounding farms — they would get her, there was no telephone to tell her in advance to get ready, you know, but they came, day or night, and when she had a nursing baby just then, she would take that along, because she never knew if she would stay only a few hours or a few days! And she took the baby along, and then sometimes she found that they ran out of food, and there was no bread any more, and she would pitch in, and she would

bake *Schnettje* (biscuits). And once she wanted to bake *Schnettje*, and didn't find any baking sheets to put them on, and when she looked through the window, she saw that the boys had tied a string to the sheets and were using it for a sleigh! and things like that, it was sometimes difficult, you know? And if she went to very poor families, sometimes they really didn't have very much nourishing food in the house, and when it was in town, she would always go back the next day to bathe the baby and bring something to eat if necessary, chicken noodle soup had been made ready, and she would take some butter, so that the sick lady would have something to put on her bread, and that kind of thing.

Once when I was, as her youngest child, was nine months old, her younger sister gave birth to twins. And her sister didn't have big girls at home, and wasn't very strong either, so she offered to take one of the twins with her and keep it for a while. So she took one of these little babies and brought it home, nursed this baby with me together for a whole year yet, then she taught this little baby to eat and brought it back to her sister.

So she's almost a sister to you, I guess!
Yes, we always call ourselves kind of our milk-sisters, we were nursing together! Yes, and she is very close to me this day yet.

You were mentioning that sometimes a baby arrived and your mother herself had just had a baby. What did she do then?
Yes, well, this is just what happened one day! My parents were living about in the middle of town, and having no telephones, there came a man from the other end of town, and asked for her help. And then he asked my dad, you know, "Where's Mrs. Reimer?" And my dad said, "Well, she's in bed, she just had a baby three days ago!" But they need help very badly. "Well," my dad said, "just go in and see what Mrs. Reimer will say." And when he came in he asked her, and she said, "Sure, I'll try to help you. But I can't walk to the other end of town. If you would get a horse and buggy so that I can drive —" And he quickly did so. In the meantime she wrapped up her little baby, and she went there and helped the lady with the birth, and after it was finished, he drove her back again, and she was all right and the other lady, too.

Did your mother continue to be a midwife all her life, or did that stop after a while?
Well, it tapered off, you know, when doctors started to come in. Eventually they built a new hospital in Steinbach, and it was opened up in 1938, and there I had my babies after that. My mother said it would be nice to come

to the hospital, and she would come with me there and we would take it easy. And that's how it came to a stop with her being a midwife.

Did she get paid for her services?
Oh yeah! She got two dollars for her service. And sometimes, when there were people that were better off, they would give her more anyway, but usually her fee was two dollars.

And then she also did the work as an undertaker. If somebody died, she was called to come over and she would bathe the person and she would help put the body into the coffin and things like that. Overall, she was quite a busy lady.

But she enjoyed that things were going ahead, you know, and eventually we drove around with the car instead of an oxcart, ja. And when she would go along with us to Winnipeg and we would drive over the Red River so nicely on the bridge, she would never fail to mention that her dad had drowned in that Red River. Yeah, and she liked to go along with us, and one day we went out cherry picking. We happened to be close to St. Anne's, and there was the sand pit close by, and I had some of my children along, and my oldest son, Menno, he had heard so much talk about this sand pit from his uncles, that they went bathing there, and he thought this was great, now he wanted to bathe in the sand pit too. And, of course, we didn't have time, we were picking cherries, I said, but eventually Grandma said, "Well, Menno, come on, let's go swimming!" And I thought, what's that, I never heard Mom could swim! She never did so, anyway. And she went to the car and took off some of her things, so that she just had her big slip on, a long one, up to the ankles, and she went into the water with Menno. He enjoyed it just tremendously, with his grandma out there, and he still remembers how her big skirt would just blow up kind of a balloon, you know, [laughs] and she would swim there and taught him how to swim. That was really something for a grandchild!

Did she talk about any babies or mothers that died in childbirth?
Yes, I think there were two mothers that died in childbirth while she was in practice. And having delivered over six hundred babies, that was very few, I would say. She talked about hard cases, where she knew it would need a lot of prayer, and she prayed and it always came out to be good, you know. But more babies died, and were delivered dead already, you know, in those days.

When you first found out you were pregnant, how did you feel?
Yes, well, I was glad, I felt quite good about it, but in those days we didn't

go and mention it to anybody right away. We kept it a secret as long as we could. Eventually they would see it, ja.

Did you think you knew enough about it, or did you feel unsure?
Well, having your mother as a midwife, I was kind of relying on her, you know? She would know what to do, and she gave a little bit of advice, not much. In those days, I don't know, things like that weren't talked too freely about, not like now.

Were there ever any things they said not to do while you were pregnant?
No, I can't remember. Except once, I remember that when I was pregnant for the first time, and we lived together on the farm with my brother, and we had a little dog, and the dog had torn up my sister-in-law's dress while it was hanging on the line, and my brother was very mad at that little dog, you know, he just took it and slayed it and while I was milking in the barn he came in with this little dog and I saw that he had really slain it and I was kind of shocked, and then my mother, when she heard about it, she said, "But Abe, you should never have done that, it could cause very much damage to the baby to see things like that!" But luckily it didn't.

And so you continued working while you were pregnant?
Yes, we were living on the farm, and we were — well, it's not that I had to do anything except that I went milking all the time, things like that, but really we did our work like usual. In those days we used to bring our milk to Steinbach to have it separated, we were living about three and a half miles from Steinbach. And then on this morning, I hadn't slept very good, and I thought, what's going on, I have pain, you know, off and on, and I told my husband, "If you meet my mother when you take the milk to Steinbach, then tell her to come over." And that's what he did, and my mother said, "Ohhh? And then you're here yet? even if Sara felt it all night already?" And well, we weren't too much alarmed yet, but then she quickly took her own horse and buggy and came over to our place, and the baby was born at suppertime. That was the first one.

What did you do with your older children while you were in labour?
We were living close to my husband's parents, and they were sent over there. And there was a little story yet, too! When our third child was born the oldest one was five. And of course he was at the grandparents' for the night. And afterwards, when we had this little baby, it was crying in the carriage, and our five-year-old son, Menno, he went to rock it quite rough, and I said, "Don't rock her so rough, she might fall out, and she could die!"

"Oh," he said, "that wouldn't matter so much, she would go to heaven, and I would just go over to grandparents' for night, and we'd have another one!" [laughs] Because that was the only time, when he could be at the grandparents' for the night, that he could remember. [laughs]

Maria Reimer

Maria (Friesen) Reimer was born in 1904 in Greenland, Manitoba, just north of Steinbach. She and her husband, Peter, had ten children.

Maria took the time to reflect back on a long life. She was willing to answer questions and to think back to her childbearing years. Our pre-interview over tea and cookies roamed over many topics, ending with her description of a "prayer call" she and a group from her church had organized. At first they met at a church at 6:30 a.m. once a week, but later they stayed at home and simply made a telephone round. It operated like a telephone tree: Maria called a member of the group, who then dialled the next number. They let the telephone ring once and hung up. The call early in the morning was a reminder for each of them to pray for the unsaved people on their list. Her description took me back to my troubled state of mind in childhood whenever the subject of salvation came up. Maria sensed my emotions. She turned to me and asked if I was happy in the Lord. Numerous feelings fought for attention as I again confronted my childhood fears. Panic, incomprehension — what must I do to be saved? If I said yes, I was happy in the Lord, what did that mean? If I said no, would I jeopardize my chances for an interview? Who did she think she was to turn the tables on me and try to interview me? After a stretched-out moment of silence I told her life was not easy for me, and escaped to my car for the trip back to Winnipeg.

Her question had disturbed me at a preconscious level. I had a busy schedule of interviews and I needed to be confident and self-assured, not digging in my psyche to explore my anxieties. I braced myself to return to her the next week. In the meantime I told myself I was no longer a vulnerable little girl who trembled with fear during fire-and-brimstone sermons. To my joy Maria had received assurance from her prayer sessions that I was living in grace. Her confidence in me and my realization that she could not turn me back into a little girl made for good rapport. Just listening to her down-to-earth style of Plautdietsch evoked warm memories.

[Translated from Plautdietsch. English terms used by Mrs. Reimer are set off by quotation marks.]

BEFORE I WAS MARRIED, I knew very little about being in the other time, how do you say it, "pregnant." When my younger siblings were born, we had to go to the neighbours', that was a big treat, and we didn't know for how long, but in the morning we would come home and there would be a baby! But when we were already engaged, my husband went to Chicago and worked there for a year, and during that time my eldest sister talked to me about other circumstances, about pregnancy. And she said too, among other things, that the baby moved, in my stomach! [laughs] And that seemed so grotesque to me, I found it so repugnant, and I thought, Oh, I am never going to get married! I would never get married! That was too terrible. And for a while I wished that Peter would never return from Chicago. But we were engaged, we had made a commitment to each other, and I knew, when he came back we would get married, but it just seemed too terrible! And so I was always between those two. I know I will have talked about it with my other sisters, about pregnancy, but this is what I remember so very clearly. And I will have, I think, talked about it with my friends, but we knew much less than what they now know from earliest childhood on! We didn't know that.

And, well, he came back in August, and on the first of November, 1924, we got married. And not even a year later, just ten and a half months later, we had a baby. And that was terrible. [laughs] I don't even know if I really want to say it or not. Not that the pregnancy was so difficult, but the birth was so difficult. Two days. And I had such long and such difficult labours. We were living on the farm then, and the doctor came. For five hours I was under chloroform, and every once in a while he would let me regain consciousness, and when the baby was finally born, everything was supposed to be just fine, but then came the most terrible part. And that was, my afterbirth was stuck. It was stuck, and the doctor put his hand in and tore it out, inch by inch. And that was very, very terrible. I screamed. The whole time. The doctor had on his white gown, but it was completely red instead of white. Yes. And the doctor said — he was an older doctor from Lorette — he said in thirty-two years this was only the second time he had encountered a case like this, that was this difficult. A bit, maybe, but not this extreme. And my mother was there, but she shouldn't have been. She screamed, too! She should not have been there. That's how I felt. And I think she felt that way, too.

At that time the doctor usually brought a scale to weigh the baby, and the mothers usually brought an old coverlet, it was nice and soft, and ripped it up for diapers, so the first little diapers were very nice and soft. And on the farm, well, we also had to get the bed ready, we would put on "rubber sheeting," but some of the poor people would use an oilcloth! They would often have an old one that they would have ready, and of course a lot of rags were used, a lot of rags. And water was of course a big thing, "a big item." We had to make sure we had water, we'd either pump it or melt snow, and heat it, and the tubs had to be ready, the containers, and everything was outside, so it had to be brought in and warmed and the stove readied so this could all be done.

And doing the laundry was of course also a big thing at that time. I have sometimes said my "profession" was [laughs] washing dishes and washing diapers! That was my "profession"! [laughs] Mind you it was a pleasure, seeing the long clothesline full of swaying laundry, it was a real joy! But in the winter it wasn't such a pleasure, we had to hang it outside and it was like boards, the sheets and the diapers, we would bring these stiff boards inside and then we'd put up a line inside and hang it up there and usually by morning it was dry, we had an oven, an "air-tight heater." We also boiled the laundry, so the stains would all come out, we boiled them on top of the cookstove, the white wash. — Yes, that's something from long ago, yes? My first three children I had at home, and the last seven were born in the hospital.

They were born at home with a doctor though, right?

Yes, yes, I yes. Not everyone could always have a doctor. I had difficult births, but the doctor was present at each birth. And frequently, too, during my pregnancies, I sensed God's nearness. When our Peter was born, between the labour pains, I suddenly saw the heavens open. There was a circle, and I could see directly into heaven! And then the other labour pains, they were also long and difficult, I saw Jesus looking down from the edge. From the place where I could see in, Jesus was looking down. And that was very joyous for me, it strengthened me, and gave me courage to push more. I was also frequently reminded of Bible verses. With Henry, I had those two boys, with those two the Lord wonderfully gave me a Bible verse, I didn't even realize that I knew it by memory: "Wir sind sein Werk geschaffen, in Christo Jesu zu guten Werken" ("For we are his workmanship, created in Christ Jesus for good works"). I didn't even know how I was supposed to apply it to the birth. But it just came to me, through and through. "Wir sind *sein* Werk geschaffen *in* Christo Jesu zu guten Werken."

Yes. Once the babies were born, [laughs] that was a very good feeling. It was just like the Bible says, you forget then, in the joy that the child has come into the world. And you know, you've experienced it too: the birth of a baby, the pregnancy and also the experience of birth, that is a "renewal experience." The person becomes renewed. Somehow it's an experience that I can't quite explain, but it is a "renewal experience." A joyous experience. Even though it was difficult, but your whole body is refreshed, renewed. And even the, how do I say it, the relationship with the husband, as if it's something completely new. And I think it's so unfortunate when women don't want to have babies. One of my daughters said to me, when Peter, my husband, had taken her with him to the hospital to see me and the baby, she said, "Oh Mom, you looked so young, and so beautiful, you looked like a queen!" [laughs] Oh my, that was very . . . And one of my daughters,when I was concerned about her having babies, because she too had difficult births, and I was so concerned about her, she said, "Mom! Look at everything that will happen if I have a baby! I'll be a mom, and Hans will be a father, he'll be a daddy. The population of the whole world changes, and I trust in heaven, too, if I have a baby. And that has to cost something. And the cost is not too high for me." It was worth it all. Well! that shut my mouth, I couldn't keep feeling so sorry for her if she had such a good attitude. Yes.

And you also had something on that paper about breast-feeding. I'm sorry [laughs] when I talk so much about the difficult part, because it is also always connected with much that is good. But breast-feeding a baby was hard for me, because I had such sore nipples, they would crack and hurt so badly. But then we always had our methods that we used, people would give me advice. One of these was, we would crack open a walnut and then tip it over them. And that seemed to heal them. There was some healing power in them, an oil or whatever, and that helped. That helped. But otherwise I really enjoyed giving my babies the breast, especially if they fell asleep during the feeding, that was very enjoyable.

Yes, there are many things that come to mind from that time, maybe not exactly the most necessary or important things to repeat, but one woman who had no children, she said, "Those women who have babies, they can sit down once in awhile, to nurse their babies, but I always have to work!" [laughs]

Yes. And what we wore when we were pregnant, well, we did make clothes especially for that, but often we would just wear a large apron. And that was supposed to hide it a bit, but it did exactly the opposite, that exactly gave it away! [laughs] "Oh, she's wearing a large apron, she must be pregnant!" [laughs] But being pregnant was kept a bit secret. Quite different from now. We kept it quiet as long as we could. And for me, and I think for other mothers, it was like that. It was a bit of a secret between me and God. Well, between me and my husband, too; other people didn't know. But it was also a bit of a secret between me and God. And it was, how should I put it, a "partnership, to fashion an immortal soul. A partnership with God." And it had a beginning, but no end. And that was important. It was very important to me.

How do you mean, "no end"?
Well, life. Life has no end, even when we die here. So the life that's inside you when you are pregnant, it has a beginning, but it will have no end. Even a baby that is never born, I mean not born alive, it had a beginning, but no end. And I think it's too bad now with the "abortions." And I think too of Mary! When the angel Gabriel was there and said that she was going to be a mother, that she would conceive Jesus, would get pregnant through the Holy Spirit, it says there, and I think it is so, how should I say it, so loving of the Saviour, of God, that he immediately told her: "There's another woman, she is pregnant, too." And possibly her mother was no longer living, but whatever it was, He reminded her: "There is another one, she is also pregnant, that's your cousin." And she got up and went there and Elizabeth was quite astonished and said, "How is it that I am worthy of this, that the mother of my Lord comes to me." Mary had borne no child yet, and she already calls her "mother," she calls her the mother of her Lord. That which will be born is already a person. That is very much against abortion, I would say.

When we were pregnant, my sisters would be concerned. I had a lot of other little children, and once my sister phoned me and said, "Marie, what are you doing?" Oh, I said, I baked bread, and fixed a spring on the screen door, so the flies wouldn't come in, it was supposed to stay closed all the time, and I had nailed the well shut — we had a well outside, where we got our water — so the children wouldn't open the trap door to look in, or fall in. Those were some of the [laughs] preparations! There was much to get ready.

We had a healthy family, we had a large, healthy family, and yet we did have a lot of illness. The children had the measles, I had pneumonia, we had the chicken pox, also diphtheria, or scarlet fever. And the worst thing we had, that lasted longest, was whooping cough. When the oldest four children had the whooping cough we had to stay up day and night when someone was coughing, because they would stop breathing. During the day I couldn't do just anything when Peter wasn't home. I did the laundry at night, so Peter could look after the children. And staying up at night because of sick or restless children, that was not, how shall I say it, yes I would get tired, but it was not an experience that made me not want the children, it was part of "the whole game," [laughs] it was a job that we did, that was also "meaningful."

We had four girls and a boy, and again four girls and a boy. Our Peter, the oldest boy, he was in between the girls, but he wanted a baby brother so badly, and when we had another baby and it was another girl, he stood next to me, he was six or seven years old, I was looking after the baby, and he asked, "Mom, will it change into a little boy yet?" He thought maybe it would become a boy! He was fifteen when his little brother was born, and he willingly took care of him, he didn't mind a bit if the girls saw him.

Yes. One time we had visitors, the children were in the other room with the guests while I was preparing food, and I heard the woman ask, "How many children do you have?" "Oh," said one of the girls, "we have seven, and then we have Peter." [laughs]

When I was expecting my tenth child, I was not happy. I already had two sons-in-law, and I thought, "Oh, what are they going to think of those old people! Now it was time for them to have babies, not for us!" But I also did not want to have a child that was not "wanted," and I prayed, and God gave me the grace. Oh I didn't tell anybody, either, and our older girls, they asked me, "Mom, what's the matter? Why are you so sad? Tell us what's the matter!" And I didn't say, I was too, how should I say, too dissatisfied, not resigned. But finally I said, "You wouldn't be happy either if I told you." Yes, I was supposed to tell them anyway. I think they had some idea already. But when I told them, they said, "Oh, but Mom, there are so many people who will love that baby!" And that gave me a lot of strength. So in that respect, I had no experience of that, that our children didn't willingly accept it. Some mothers had it very hard that way, but I didn't.

And I said, during the months that I was carrying him, I wanted to learn what I was supposed to learn, and if this last one — I didn't know of course if this was the last one — I said to God, He should teach me whatever it was He wanted to teach me through this. And then it occurred to me, and I am sure it was from God, I was to pray for other women who were pregnant. I did that for many a woman. She wouldn't know that I was praying for her, but I was, and also for her birth, because I had had it so hard. And that's still my job. [laughs] I haven't maybe always done it, but many, many times it occurs to me, and I do it gladly. I do it gladly.

And my husband was very understanding, he had authority over me, but sometimes I thought, Oh, if only he could understand me a bit better! He had authority over me, but if only he could understand me better! But what can you expect from a man who has never been pregnant? Or has never been a woman? And a woman is built differently. I sometimes think a woman should not expect too much from a man. She can love him, be submissive to him, and make him happy, but she should not expect too much. If she feels she has to pour out her heart, she has to do that with another woman, a trustworthy, devout woman, and they can understand each other better. That's how I often thought over the years. And that is what I have also experienced.

How did you make a living in Steinbach?
My husband had a small bargain store, Reimer's Bargain Store. He sold small items, also second-hand goods, a bargain store, and we were able to live off it. And we had a big garden, a very big garden, and the children worked in it. In summer we had raspberries which we sold, and Peter would also take them to Winnipeg, to the hospitals. I would sometimes go along with him to the hospitals, and as far as I could tell, they bought great quantities. I even saw the sisters in the St. Boniface Hospital cutting up beans for canning. And when the children were old enough, the oldest girls started too. At that time there was a great shortage of teachers, and they could already start teaching with grade eleven — they never taught in Steinbach, not those children. But they found employment, and brought their money home. But then later they did finish high school. Some continued going to school after that, some attended Bible School.

That was a busy time!
Very busy. Very busy. I did all my own sewing for the children. I made coats and shoes, everything myself. I didn't always make everything, but the clothes yes. And always in autumn it was time to make decisions. Some mothers would tell me their children did not want to go to school, and I said for us it's that they all want to go! And then decisions had to be made, whether one would stay home or another, who would stay home. So they would discuss it and say, when Mother does the laundry, then this or that one will stay home. And when Father goes to Winnipeg to make purchases for the store, it would be this or that one, usually it was the same one who would work in the store.

Could you tell me something about your wedding? A bride would wear a dark dress at that time, right?

Yes. Well, my dress was what they called "sandalwood." I had red hair! [laughs] And the wedding was in autumn. I sewed my own dress. My wedding took place on the farm. My husband's parents had quite a big house, and the wedding was in the house. There were about a hundred people. We were married by Father's very good friend, Heinrich Dyck. They came by horse from Kleefeld across the field, a huge hay field, to the farm at Prairie Rose, to marry us. And they stayed for night, we were all at the parents' place for night. And the text for the service was Romans 12:12. That is something I will never forget, it was: "Seid fröhlich in Hoffnung, geduldig in Trübsal, haltet an am Gebet" ("Rejoice in your hope, be patient in tribulation, be constant in prayer"). And that was very useful to me.

Elizabeth Krahn

Elizabeth Krahn was born in 1953 in Winnipeg. She and her former husband, Jamie Marrin, have three children. Elizabeth has integrated bachelor of science social work training with macrobiotic counselling, and more recently with Reiki, and is currently applying the latter in the field of gerontology.

Darlene Birch, a traditional lay midwife in Winnipeg, supplied me with Elizabeth's name because Elizabeth had given birth in her own home recently. Elizabeth was the first younger woman I interviewed, and she revealed the gap between the generations. She grew up in Canada as the youngest child in a family that emigrated from Russia in the 1940s. She spoke eloquently of the differences between her immigrant parents' attitude to modern medicine and her own.

There is a contrast between the stories of the older women who gave birth at home and the accounts of the younger women's modern home births. For the older women it was a sign of progress to be able to have one's babies in a hospital (although Margaret Sawatzky questioned the idea of leaving one's comfortable home at a time when it would be so much more relaxing to stay in it). By contrast, the young women who chose to give birth at home in the eighties had often had a bad first birth experience in a hospital and hoped a home birth would be a less intrusive event, with fewer interventions. The ones I spoke to made this decision after much consideration.

I WANTED TO EXPERIENCE AS NATURAL a birthing process as possible, and so my focus was on having the child at home, although this wasn't possible for the first baby, because the doctor I was seeing at the time, who was willing to do home births, was not willing to do a first birth at home. Throughout the pregnancy we read a lot about birthing procedures and the breathing techniques, like Lamaze, and I have some books about birthing in other cultures, in traditional cultures, and so we really became well versed on the subject. I haven't read a thing, I don't think, since that first birth, but we wanted to be well prepared, and a lot of the knowledge that used to be given via mother and grandmother is something that we now have to read about, because it's been lost or discouraged. Both my grandmothers died before I was born, and my mother wasn't really — I guess was a bit apprehensive about talking about these matters, and so we never really talked much about menstruation and birthing and that sort of thing.

Did she have her children in hospitals in Russia?
I think she had at least one of them at home, and the others in hospitals. But I don't recall what her experience was with the home birth, and who would have been there. I suppose it would have been a midwife, I'm sure there would have been women who were able to do that at the time, but her feeling always was that it was much safer to do it in the hospital. Although later, I'm told, when there was a lot of illness going around, the hospital was the last place you wanted to take your sick child, because they would die there, being exposed to a lot of illness. That was in Russia.

So going back to your birth experiences then.
OK. I'll talk a little bit about the first birth, which happened in the hospital with a doctor who was familiar with home births. I found that although he promised that I wouldn't be encouraged to take medication and so on, the nurses convinced me that I could. He said that if I was feeling a little tense or if things were difficult, I could take Demerol if I wanted, and I thought, well, maybe if it will relax me, maybe I should. Somehow I had a real need to — I wasn't in complete ownership of my birth, and I felt somehow that I had to prove to this man that I could have a good, natural birth, or else he wouldn't do any home births for me later on. And so I wasn't as relaxed with the birth as I had wanted to be. My water didn't break, my cervix wasn't dilating enough, and so I had some difficulty. He almost convinced me I needed a Caesarean, and so he kind of went in the completely opposite direction with me! Thank goodness I didn't need a Caesarean, he allowed me to go through the birth, and after about twelve hours I had a boy! So the first birthing experience could have been a lot worse, but it certainly had its

negative points to it. With subsequent births, having the children at home, I felt much more relaxed. By the time I had the next child, I had met a midwife who was willing to come and help me with the birth, so that birth went very smoothly, and I had no trouble dilating, I was comfortable, I was in my own home, my husband was there. My husband was there for the first birth as well, but the nurses convinced me not to listen to him. He kept saying, "Don't take any medication, just relax," and the nurses said, "He's not having the baby! Do what you want to do!" So they weren't very helpful, although they thought they were.

You were sort of torn between all this conflicting advice.
That's right. And I was convinced before going to the hospital that this wasn't going to happen to me, I was prepared for this to happen, and I wasn't going to go along with it. But once I was there, it wasn't very easy to live up to. I'd had false labour the week before, I'd already been there one night the week before, and here I was again, and this was — with the first birth, you know, I wasn't really sure exactly how the labour would feel. I'm very easily influenced by other people's impressions of what's happening to me, and so I wasn't sure that I knew what was supposed to be happening myself, exactly.

Would you like to describe one of the other births, the home births?
I'll describe the second one, because the contrast between the first and second one was quite great. With Annalies, I went to bed one evening, and woke up at one o'clock, the mucus had popped, and I thought, Oh, I'm in labour! and then I went back to sleep, and probably had contractions throughout the night, and by the morning when I woke up they were fairly strong. I phoned the midwife about nine and I said, "Whenever you get here will probably be fine." She got there around eleven. By that time I was in pretty strong labour, and I had her by one o'clock. The feeling of actually having her coming out was such a contrast from having Brian come out, because I wasn't feeling a lot with Brian, except the awareness of pushing, but with Annalies it was like — all of a sudden she was just coming out, and with one push she was there! And also this incredible stretching, that wasn't the greatest feeling, but it's wonderful to know that you can have a birth completely on your own, and that your body is well equipped to do it, and that if you're in tune with your body and allowing *it* to do all the work, then you have nothing to fear. As long as everything is in good working order. So then it's my job to keep it in good working order by appropriate diet and appropriate exercise and the ability to listen to what it's telling me. And this is what brings me back to traditional birthing, that women were

able to do this much more in the past, and we need to relearn that skill. We have to do it intellectually to begin with, but then incorporate that into our intuitive knowledge.

Is there something about a hospital that encourages you not to depend on yourself?
I have a good example from a book by Ivan Illich. He describes a situation in Third World countries where women used to be able to have their children quite successfully at home without any help at all, and with the advent of hospitals in these parts of the world, and, say the Americans, or whoever it may be, pushing hospitals and public health upon people, women completely lost their confidence in having their children at home, and birthing became almost an illness, or something that required going to the hospital to do, and so it was completely out of their hands. And this is what's happened to us here, we feel that when we're pregnant, we're really out of touch with what's happening inside of us, we're completely in the hands of doctors, who tend to use a lot of equipment on us, and tend to prefer a lot of measures that can actually be detrimental to the health of the child.

Can you remember what started you on the idea of home births? Did you know of other people who had them?
I'm not even sure how that started, except to say that my husband and I tend — in the political jargon — to be anarchists. We tend to prefer a lifestyle that does not lean heavily on modern systems, and does not support the continuation of modern systems that are abusive, or rely a lot on professionals.

Someone mentioned recently that there was a strong spiritual element in birth. Did you feel that?
With the first birth I was in the hospital overnight. I went home the next morning, so I wasn't there long. I was very tired, and much groggier, I was much less alert, probably. With my second one — my mother was appalled — she came over a few hours later, and I was going up and down the stairs between the third floor and basement, because the washroom was downstairs, and she told me how when she was in Russia, they were told to lie flat in bed for two weeks and they had to wear some kind of stiff material around their abdomen for a couple of weeks, so that the uterus would go back in, and she was just appalled. But I was quite ready for company. My mother-in-law arrived from Toronto one hour after the birth, and was very pleased to see the baby right there waiting for her, and other people dropped in. So "spiritual" to me can include that, I guess. I've heard people say that during their birth experience they feel connected to all mothers of the past and the

present, and they have this profound sense of connection with motherhood. I didn't really have that kind of a feeling, although I have a small feeling like that. Shortly after Brian's birth I had an overwhelming sense of motherhood that comes to you after your first child, that this is now a child who will be with you for the rest of your life, or with you in spirit, anyway, and this responsibility that you now carry in and of itself does an awful lot to your self-image.

The birth at home of my second child was wonderful for Brian, too, who was two and a half at the time. I can still see his face when he saw her for the first time, and his eyes lit up. He was really waiting for this baby and wanted five more when he saw her! It's really important for the bonding of the children to be able to have the baby there from the beginning, and not experience a separation from the mother. Because then sometimes you have this feeling from the older child that now the younger one is with the mother. The mother is away for five days in the hospital with this other baby, and then when Mother comes home with the baby, they don't really want the baby. And it's a much stronger sense of separation from the mother. This doesn't always have to happen, but certainly with my first two at that point there was a strong connection. And they were both nursing at the same time! He started nursing even more, because he was reminded of the fact that newborns nurse every two hours — he had had the nursing just going to bed, and now he started nursing every two hours, and of course the milk supply was gushing in, so he was quite pleasantly surprised by that.

What were the reactions to your having a home birth?

I can't really recall a response from friends. My mother was probably concerned. The rest of my family may have been concerned, but they were — covering up a bit more, perhaps. And as with some of the other choices that I make in my life, my mother worries that I'm denying my children certain basic needs. So there was a concern that if something happened, what would you do? And in this country, where all this professional help is available, why would you deny this to your child? But she also knows that I will continue to do what I choose, and that I'll do it to the best of my ability, and so she lets me know what her concern is, and then she kind of tries to live with my choice. [laughs]

Last week we talked a little bit about your place in the family as the youngest child in a big family. Could you talk about that?

Sure. What was aroused after Brian's birth was a memory of my own childhood, being the youngest and often feeling left out of things, not being adult enough to participate in certain conversations, or to be deemed worthy of having an opinion, or always having the plastic plate because dishes only came in sets of six, and I was the seventh, [laughs] having the little spoon, that sort of thing. And now having a child that was several years younger than all the other grandchildren, of which there are quite a few, I experienced some pain, just knowing that he might experience some pain, or feel that he wasn't quite fitting in. And when I began to attend family gatherings with him, as an infant, people showed a lot of interest in him, but they had become so used to all the children and all the men and all the women going off somewhere and doing whatever they did, that somehow this baby didn't have anywhere to fit in. And so I found myself, one Easter, alone with Brian in the living room! All the various groups were doing something, and I felt left out.

What other memories or feelings about your ancestors came back to you when you became a mother?

I think after I began to have children I became more and more interested in learning about my roots, in having an awareness of where the family came from and particularly wanting to know who my maternal grandmother was. My mother had told me many things about her childhood, but one of her real lacks was that her mother died when my mother was eight. She hadn't ever really known her that well, because it was quite a large family, and she has no picture of her either, so she has a sense of grief when it comes to her mother. And I'm sure I pick this up. I seem to have a strong need to know who she was, and what she was about, and what kind of strengths she carried. And I almost felt at one point that maybe I was her, you know, that the spirit of my grandmother was touching me somehow, and this leads me to my question today: What do we carry in our lives that may have been begun in the hearts of our parents or our grandparents? What kind of work are we doing in this life that they fed into, that they started, perhaps?

You've heard stories about her that give you very vivid images of her, though, do you not?

My mother tells me a story of when they lived on a farm, and two or three men came to raid whatever they had in the barn. And my grandmother heard somebody out there and went out — my mother seems to remember the scene. And perhaps she was carrying another baby or something. So here were these men with guns or whatever, and my grandmother, looking very stern, yelling at them. And finally one of the men said to the one with the gun, "Can't you see that she has little children? Leave her alone!" And then they left. But the image that this gives me is one of real strength, and so whenever I am in a moment of weakness I like to think about my grandmother, because I feel that she has something to offer me. I need to be called to a place of strength.

Part of our Mennonite heritage has been hearing the stories of suffering, especially in Russia. Could you talk about that?
Yes, I remember as a child hearing a lot of stories from my mother about her childhood, and when I think of it now, it must have been important for her to do this, because she's the only one of her family that was able to come to Canada. In many ways she must have felt very alone, very separated from her family. And so she found that I was the one that listened to her, and she could tell me all these things. But the stories that she told me were all very sad stories, there weren't many happy memories. I think the only happy memory was when somebody got a candy for Christmas or for their birthday, and they separated it eight different ways or something like that. But the stories that I remember were ones of death, when people died and how they died and why they died. The one I remember in particular was three little boys, who were all born before she was, they were gone before she was born, but they died in two weeks of diphtheria. One of them might have been a baby, the others might have been two and four, something like that. And then there were others in the family as well that died at different times, an eighteen-year-old son who died of typhoid fever. My grandmother had a total of twelve children, and I believe only five of them reached adulthood.

Did these stories mean more to you later in life?
Well, when I began to have my own children and recalled the stories of my grandmother, I began to really feel the pain that she must have felt, and I wondered how, having lost that many children, she could have the strength to have more, or to live through her life, knowing that any of her other children could die at any point because of the conditions there. She died at forty-three or something, she'd had typhoid fever. I'm not sure if that's exactly why she died, but that combined with hunger, there'd been a famine I think, in 1919 or '20, and she died not long after that. And so when I think of how I felt carrying a child to term and then actually birthing a child and thinking, How can I ever love another child as much as I love the first one! And then thinking to myself, How can I ever yell at this child! And then finding that, sure enough, when they get to be a little bit older, you do yell at them — but you've had that experience of wondering, how could I ever do it? Then how could you ever watch the child die, and then have more children, and not feel a lot of pain and a lot of — what's the word, a

lot of fear about their lives. I can just imagine the amount of grief that she must have carried.

Does the Mennonite community or church still have some meaning for you?
Well, I no longer attend the Mennonite church. I felt that I wasn't experiencing what the Scriptures were really talking about, I didn't feel the heart in it, and so I left the church, and found some heart in different places. But what I feel about my Mennonite roots is strong. I feel that with any spiritual group there is a real excitement, a real spiritual yearning when that group is formed, that there is a real life and vitality there, and then after some time it can become lost. It may not be gone forever, it may still be there somewhere for people to find, but it's not necessarily easy to find, and I certainly wasn't experiencing it. But I know that part of that life, which the Mennonites expressed in the form of community and in the form of pacifism and peace, those things I'm very drawn to, and I look for ways of expressing, and for ways of experiencing more fully. Not just in having "peace not war," but in truly being peaceful with myself, and in being able to trust my neighbour, in being able to live in close proximity with other people, and perhaps even share housing with people, and not get into daily squabbles and tensions, being able to work through those in a peaceful way. So truly bringing these ideals into my practical, day-to-day life. And also fitting those within the larger perspective of God, and the divine, and sort of the larger picture.

But you mentioned something earlier that I want to comment on. You mentioned the fact that because of the conditions that our grandparents lived in in the early 1900s, and the epidemics and various famines and so on, that the next generation felt very pleased to be able to have hospitals and to be able to have their children in hospitals and so on. And I just wanted to mention that often people feel that hospitals are more civilized and more help is available to us if there are hospitals, but it's only in contrast to really awful conditions, such as famines and the epidemics. Now those things happened because the early 1900s were a bad scene in Russia. There was the revolution, and there were wars, and various things happening. So those weren't ideal conditions. And if you talk traditional diet, what they were experiencing at that time was not the traditional diet at its best. That was traditional diet at its worst. And so of course the hospital is going to look very welcoming after something like that. This is the difficulty I suppose I have in relating to my mother, who experiences everything today as being such an improvement over all the awful things that happened in her childhood, and what we need to look at is even further back, to when life was happening in more harmony, and what people were doing then, when everything was in a healthier state, when there was peace, and when people were growing food, and people weren't starving, when things were available, when their environment was not being destroyed by war and whatever the case may be. And so these are the things that make for health and that make for healthy births.

Evelyn Rempel Petkau

Evelyn (Rempel) Petkau was born in Winnipeg in 1953 and has lived in Washington, D.C., and Elkhart, Indiana, as well as several places in Manitoba. At the time of the interview she lived in Carman, in southern Manitoba. She and her husband, Brian, have three children. Evelyn and Brian lived in Elkhart while they attended the Associated Mennonite Biblical Seminaries. She worked as a Mennonite Central Committee voluntary service social worker in Washington, D.C.

Evelyn opened my eyes to the world of women who were claiming their own power, just as Maria Reimer showed me how older women were grounded in their strength and wisdom.

The highlight of my interview with Evelyn was the story of the home birth in 1986 of her son, Justin, her third child. She told her story effortlessly and musically as she nursed her son and refereed disputes among her children, thus putting birth squarely in the context of daily life. I left her house feeling blessed.

Our oldest daughter was born in Goshen, Indiana, in 1980, and I had quite a routine kind of experience with the pregnancy and delivery of her. It seemed like a very short pregnancy, because I only found out after I was about three and a half months pregnant, and because we weren't expecting the child at all, it was a surprise. At that time already I was exploring some alternatives. When I found out I was pregnant it was like stepping out into something completely new. We had discussed having children, but not the planning and the preparation for it, and that kind of thing. But I knew, and Brian knew, too, that it was something we both wanted to be very involved in, to make the choices our choices, that sort of thing. So we checked out doctors, and we chose to have a doctor in Goshen rather than in Elkhart, because in Goshen there seemed to be more openness. But they wouldn't permit us to use the birthing room, because it was our first child. And so we just accepted that. I went through my labour in the birthing room, kind of hoping that things would work out that I could just stay there, but in the end we had to go to the delivery room, and I stayed my three days in the hospital, and then we were discharged, and everything went very smoothly. It was an eight-hour labour, and most of that I spent at home. I wasn't in a hurry to get to the hospital, to go through it there.

Our second daughter was born in Altona two years later, in 1982, and there our options were more limited. There was no birthing room, you went the structured route, and if there were concerns, or anything that placed anyone at any kind of high risk, you were automatically sent to Winkler or Winnipeg, the hospital wasn't equipped to work with anything more involved. So we checked with the doctor beforehand whether we could have the baby in the hospital and then be discharged immediately. And he was really reluctant to do that. We also asked him if Brian could catch the baby, and that was out of the question, he gave a definite no to that. The doctor said he wasn't even allowed to catch his own children when they were born. But he didn't say a definite yes or no that I could be discharged the day that she was born. As it turned out our doctor was on holidays at the time of her birth, so we used a different doctor, and after she was born, I asked if I could go home, and he said, "Well, what did the other doctor say?" and we said, well, he hadn't said that we couldn't, so kind of by default we were able to go home. But it was surprising to a lot of people. Several people went to the hospital to visit me there, and found that I wasn't there. It was a kind of unfamiliar experience to them. [laughs]

What other repercussions were there because you chose to go home early?
Well, it seemed like a big inconvenience to the hospital in many ways, because usually the public health nurse comes to visit you, and makes a record of the baby's birth, and then they know how to follow up with immunization and home visits and that kind of thing, and that didn't happen, that didn't follow its "natural" course. Sort of threw a hitch into, or made it a little less convenient for them. The message that came through was: You'll regret this later on, because you aren't giving yourself the rest you need and the care you need, and it'll catch up with you. — We are so

set in our way of doing things, and assume that that is the only way of doing things, and then when you choose to do something differently, you have to take that whole responsibility on yourself, for whatever happens, regardless of whether it was as a result of what you did, or whether it would have happened. That's what we found with Justin's birth, too. When you make your own choices, your own decisions, and they go contrary to the way most people do, you are given a greater burden of responsibility for your choices, and so you hope things will work out well.

Earlier you mentioned that some of your experiences as a social worker in Washington left a lasting impression. Could they have influenced you in choosing home birth?
Yes. We lived there for two years before we had any children, and I worked with a lot of lower-class families, mostly black women, who were single parents. There was a hospital in the inner city where most of these women were referred to because they catered more to the lower class, that was where they were situated and that was primarily their clientele. What was so shocking was to learn that fifty percent of the births there were Caesarean sections. I remember going there with them and feeling the fear with them, but not being able to prepare them, and feeling like I couldn't even give them moral support and the ammunition to be able to stand up for themselves there. There were a lot of student doctors who did their training there, and these women were without spouses, they were without anybody to speak for them, and it was such a feeling of helplessness and loss of control. And even though I wasn't giving thought at that time to having children and what I would do, I remember feeling very angry at that whole situation. Some of these mothers had had quite a number of births already, and they were saying to these women, if you've had three C-sections, you can't have any more, and so making those kinds of decisions for them as well.

What did they have to do then?
They had to have their tubes tied, or that sort of thing. But in that city, where there is so much diversity, we were also exposed to home births and very short hospital stays, six hours or whatever, and that really widened my understanding and my knowledge of births, and so I think I had more options open to me. If I had just grown up in Altona, say, I don't know if I would have done the same thing.

So for your third baby you chose home birth.
Yes. As soon as we knew that we were expecting Justin, who was born in

1986, we really felt that that was the route we wanted to go. I guess I should speak for myself: I really felt that was what I wanted to do. I remember after Tamara was born, we felt our family was big enough, and I mentioned sometime in the course of a conversation with my mother that probably we wouldn't have any more children. She sounded disappointed and surprised, and just off the top of my head I said, not unless there was nuclear disarmament, world nuclear disarmament, or I could have a home birth [laughs] would I have another baby. So as soon as we found out that we were expecting Justin, I was eager to pursue that, and Brian went along with me, he didn't object at all. I think he would have probably more quickly, at that time, chosen to go the hospital route, I think he had more apprehensions, at least initially. Now I don't think he would.

What prompted you, had you heard of other home births?
I had heard of other home births. I don't know if I knew of any one person in my generation that had a baby at home. But I had read about them, and I think I had heard of them through the La Leche League. My hospital experiences weren't negative experiences. I think the only negative part of them was that I felt things were out of my control. Fortunately for me, my pregnancies and deliveries were very normal, and went very well, and quickly. So it wasn't like there was a lot of intervention. But it felt like my decisions were all made for me, and anything that I would want that was out of the ordinary was out of my control. I think also part of it was that the whole birth experience is so special, I mean there's no other event in life that really measures up to that. And we wanted to keep it special, and somehow when you go through the routine, and you go through your ten-minute visits to the doctor, and that kind of thing, it minimizes the whole thing. And I guess part of it was just that — it's like a wedding. You want to personalize that experience, you want to do more than just streamline your whole process.

How did you go about arranging for a home birth?
A woman I met at a La Leche League meeting referred me to a woman in Winnipeg who had just had a home birth. She turned out to be a Mennonite woman too. I met with her and she gave me the names of three midwives. Two of them didn't really like to go out of the city very much, so I phoned the third midwife, Darlene Birch, and she was very willing right from the start.

And did you have a doctor too?
Yes, I already had contacted a doctor. At my first appointment with him I

had asked if he would be willing to come and help deliver our baby at home. He had a student doctor with him at the time, and they were both so stunned, they didn't know how to respond, because I don't think they had had to deal with that question before, it just caught them off guard. I remember them looking at each other and then sort of hemming and hawing, and trying to say things that would make me change my mind, and then saying, "Well, no, I would give you back-up services if you needed them, but I don't think I could do that." Which was what I expected to hear, but I wanted him to know what I was pursuing, and I still wanted to follow through with prenatal care, because if I needed him in the end, he would be familiar with what we had experienced.

So you saw a doctor and a midwife. Are there any differences in their approach to pregnancy?

Yes, yes. The visits were so different. I would wish for every woman a visit like the ones we experienced with the midwife. With my doctor it was in and out of his office in a matter of minutes, and he just did the very routine things, your blood pressure, feeling the position of the baby, charting your weight, measuring you, listening to the baby's heartbeat, and that's about it. Asking how are you, and giving me a chance if I had any questions to raise them, but it was very quick and very matter-of-fact. And the other day I heard that doctors are paid a very small fee through Medicare for all the prenatal visits and the delivery in normal sorts of circumstances. It isn't worth their while to spend more time with the mother, they aren't paid for any of the extras, unless there are major complications, like a C-section, or something like that. So there's no incentive for them to treat you otherwise. Whereas with my midwife, I guess half the time we came to her place and half the time she came to our place for the visits, and no visit was under two hours. Mind you, there's a lot of visiting, but that also helped to give you the time to get to know each other and ask a lot of questions that we might not otherwise have asked. And the other really neat part of that was, the whole family was involved. When she would go to do the physical checkup part of it, usually the girls were right there on the bed with me, and she would take a doll and she would lay the doll on the top of my tummy to show them the position that the baby was in. They were very much aware of what was going on. So that was really good. Whereas otherwise I went by myself to see the doctor, and it was just a conversation between him and myself. The rest of the family, the children especially, were very distant from what was happening. And then there were occasions, one or two times, where I really appreciated having both of them check out. Towards the end of the pregnancy, about the seventh month, when I had my visit with the doctor, he noted that there was no weight gain on the baby's part, or no growth on the baby's part, which really concerned him, and so he recommended that I go for an ultrasound. And his concern got me quite concerned and worried, but I asked him, well just how safe is an ultrasound? And he said, well it hasn't been around long enough for us to really know, in the long range, whether there are any effects, or side effects or anything like that for ultrasound, but it has been tested on — mice, I think he said, and there were no effects that would cause any concern, no effects at all. Well, that really helped to make up my mind that I didn't want to do that if I had any option not to, because if he couldn't give me any more of a definite — what I wanted to hear from him was that we are 100 percent sure that there are no ill effects. So when I got home I phoned Darlene and asked her, and she asked me a lot of questions that he never seemed to consider, that he never discussed with me. For example, what had been my weight gain, and my weight gain had been considerable, more than in the past. And then she said that usually it takes one or two weeks for the baby to take on that weight gain that you take on. Darlene said that if I wanted to give myself another week and see what happened, probably some of that weight would be transferred to the baby. And the other thing she said was the position the baby is in. The doctor determines the size by making that measurement, and if the baby is leaning to one side the measurement won't be as great as if the baby's back is right in the middle. So if the baby's position has changed, it will be different, too, and could well be less than before. Darlene came out, and sure enough, the baby had fallen to one side sort of, so it was off centre, and she was just so reassuring. I phoned the doctor and told him that we had decided not to have an ultrasound. In the end, when Justin was born, he was nine pounds five ounces, so there certainly didn't need to be concern about his weight gain.

What about your friends and parents and acquaintances, what was their response to your wanting a home birth?
Well, negative. [laughs] We didn't tell many people, because we didn't know until the end, either, what would happen. When I asked the doctor initially whether he would deliver the baby at home, he said no, when I returned a month later for my next appointment, he said yes, he would! He had given it considerable thought, and he would do that. And then when I returned a month later, for my next appointment, he said no, he had discussed it with his colleagues and with the College of Physicians and Surgeons, and they had discouraged him, they would not back him up, and he said he did not have the portable equipment he would need to do that. So he declined then. My parents were overseas and they wouldn't be back before his birth,

and I had written them after he had said yes, that my doctor had said he would attend the birth. When I learned otherwise, I never wrote them back to say that no, he had changed his mind, so we just never really talked about it further till after the birth. Somehow Brian's parents learned about it before Justin was born, and were very concerned and upset, it was very hard for them. To this day they call Justin a miracle baby.

Were their experiences bad, or do you know why they were so concerned?
Well, both my mother and Brian's mother don't remember their birthing experiences, the actual birth of their children, because they weren't conscious. They had been, I think, led to believe that it is awful, that it is so painful, how can you stand to be awake and aware during that time. And when I listened to them tell me some of their experiences, I realized that they were put out just after they had experienced all the pain. It's at that point that they are put out, or put under, and they didn't have any coaching, they didn't have anyone present to help them through the labour, through the difficult and more painful times. And so sure, it was awful, not knowing what was going on, and being isolated from people that care about you. So I can understand how they feel.

Right from the beginning when we made the decision to try and pursue a home birth, we did that purely as a personal decision. It was something we realized we wanted, and not that we felt anybody else should want or wish for. We could very much understand the feelings of other people, but we wanted that freedom for ourselves to make that choice. We didn't talk about it at any length with anybody other than the midwife, of course, and only after Justin was born, we began to feel the repercussions. The relationship with the doctor just went cold, really cold, and other people, especially nurses, who were friends, didn't understand, and I think the response was anger when there wasn't understanding. But it was interesting, there were a number of people who came to visit me, especially some older women, and unsolicited, told me their birthing experiences. They were probably more accepting of it, I'm not sure why — almost as though they had a feeling maybe that something had been taken away from them at one time — and also I guess because it opened something up. It was something we could talk about because it was different, it wasn't just a routine kind of thing. So there were different responses, but by far the majority of the people that we knew and encountered did not understand, really.

So what was the experience then, the home birth; what happened?
Oh, it was just — I'd repeat the experience again, it was very special. Justin was born later than his due date, and as the waiting got on, Brian became

quite concerned that things would run smoothly. It was spring, and Darlene lived two hours away, and what if it stormed and she couldn't make it, and that kind of thing. We had talked all this over with Darlene, and she had left her oxygen tank at our place and a very nice simple manual that's written up for taxi-cab drivers, you can make very quick reference to whatever section you need. And he had reviewed that and reviewed that. [laughs]

As it turned out, Justin was born in the middle of the night. My water broke around midnight and we phoned Darlene right away, but I almost felt like telling her, take your time, my water has just broken, nothing else has happened, don't feel that you have to rush or anything. But she said she was leaving right away, so in two hours we could expect her. For the first hour we just got things ready, we sterilized the things that she had left for us and hauled a mattress onto the living room floor and got things ready. An hour later I started to have contractions, and they were extremely strong contractions, and just minutes apart. When the labour pains came, I went to lie down on the bed. I was very uncomfortable, it just didn't feel like a good position, and when his head crowned, it was the first time, actually in all my birthing experiences, that I felt I didn't have control of my breathing, and I thought, this is too much, in fifteen minutes from nothing to his head crowning, there must have been a lot of muscle working there. If I had pushed, he would have been born at that time, but I just didn't have an urge to push, and then I felt the baby coming back up, going back in. And then Brian suggested that I get up and walk around, and so I did. We went downstairs and —

You went down the stairs?! [laughs]

Oh yes, [laughs] and just walked. Walked and walked. And every time a contraction came, I clung to him, and then walked again. We had a small house, and it was getting so that I could barely do one circle and the next contraction would come. So they were very, very frequent, and poor Brian was trying between these contractions to get everything ready, he was really scrambling, and looking at his watch, I hadn't realized he was doing that, he told me later on, he had a sense the baby was going to be born before Darlene was there, so he was quite nervous. And I can remember finally feeling I couldn't even walk any more, and so what I did was I just leaned over the chesterfield, got down on my knees and leaned over on the chesterfield, that felt like what I needed to do. And he was rubbing my back, and he had this little taxi-cab's manual in his lap that he was flipping through as he was rubbing my back, and it really felt like the baby was going to be born, and he said, "Hold on!" [laughs] "Twenty more minutes, hold on!" [laughs] And the head popped out. I didn't push or anything. I guess Justin just really wanted to be born, because I never once pushed for him to come out, and another contraction and his body came out, and Brian said it was just so slippery, he just felt like it was very, very slippery, and so he was born just like that, and I remember just holding him, his cord was still attached and still inside me, and we were just looking at him, and it must have been several seconds later that one of us asked, is it a boy or a girl, nothing mattered, it was just that here was this living, breathing human being, and then, the way the cord sort of came down between his legs, it wasn't easily apparent what sex he was. And then Brian went and woke our daughters. We had thought that they would probably be awake for some of the labour, we anticipated a longer labour, and they would each have jobs to do. We had ice ready in the freezer, and one of them would give me ice and another one would get the towels and everything, so the first thing they did in their state of semi-sleep, it was about 2:20 or so, was they went to do their jobs. [laughs] And then they came and held him, and they were so excited, they didn't go back to sleep until about 6:30 in the morning.

And when did Darlene arrive?

Twenty minutes after he was born. So we just sat there in the living room and held him, and didn't do anything, we just waited, and then Darlene walked in and she said, "Oh, he's a big boy!" And then she checked everything out for us. It seems to me it was almost an hour when she said finally that I should try and push the afterbirth out. And for that I had to really push, I guess my body thought it had finished its work, but that came, and she examined that, it was a very healthy placenta. We kept the placenta. I don't know how it would sound to many people, but we saved it, we froze it and we thought that we would plant it with a tree somewhere, do something significant with it. And then after that she ran the bath water for me, and cleaned up everything, and gave me the baby in the bath tub, and Justin and I just were together. In the hospital you're told not to get the baby's umbilical cord wet, you just sort of sponge-bathe the baby. But she said that swabbing the umbilical cord with alcohol is not necessary, so we never did it, and it fell off a lot sooner and healed really well. So you wonder why they recommend such different kind of care in looking after it.

And then Justin and I went upstairs to bed. We had decided ahead of time what music we wanted, we listened to Pachelbel's Canon in D. That day still stands out in my mind as being a very special day. Later on our children went out to play, it was a very nice day, a spring day, and we were told later on by the neighbours that there was a whole bunch of children, and they had all been singing "Away in a Manger" most of that day. This was spring, it was quite a bit after Christmastime! [laughs]

Brian too was very tired, so he came up to bed with us after a while, and two times we kind of woke up and here were at least seven or eight children just standing over us. The girls had led them into the house to come and see the baby and us, and here were all these big eyes, and they were so quiet, they were just standing, and looking at Justin, and then they would quietly traipse out, and then the second time a slightly different group, some new children and some of the same children came and took a look at him and then went back down. It was just such a good day, I think we will always remember that day as being very special. Just as the other births were, too, but very different kinds of memories related to that.

What type of follow-up did Darlene Birch give?
She made several visits to our home, and sometimes she brought her whole family, or part of her family, and sometimes she came by herself. Her follow-up was as comfortable and as thorough as the prenatal visits were, and I really appreciated those lengthy visits again. In many ways it felt like she was my mother, you know, that all the questions you had, all the uncertainties you had, there was a place to take them and to bounce them off and that kind of thing. Whereas with the doctor it was your regular six-week checkup, and that was about it, and then your baby has the ongoing six-month and twelve-month kind of follow-up. I have always felt, although I haven't seen Darlene for a long time, that she is available to me, if I needed her.

What is there about the philosophy of midwifery, in your experience, that's different from going to a doctor?
I think largely, for one thing, that the whole childbirth process is a very natural process, it's not like a pathology, which the doctors' approach seems to treat it as. The other thing that we really felt with Darlene was that I was in control, that I was the one that was making the choices and doing the work, and that she was there to assist me. I remember when she arrived right after his birth, and Brian said something about his involvement, and she in a very gentle way reminded him that I had delivered the baby. [laughs] That really struck Brian, he probably won't ever forget that. In a very gentle way putting the mother in full charge, and yet with all the back-up and the resources there, and that it's a very natural course of events and also that the woman follows her intuitions, there are no set guidelines.

It sounds ideal.
It was.

If you knew someone who was pregnant now, would you advise them to do the same?

I would like to, there's that part of me that would say, I had a really good experience with my home birth and would recommend it to anybody, but I haven't. There have been one or two women that have called me, and when they approach me, then I do, when the question becomes theirs. But because of the response I got to our experience, I know that many times that would be a turn-off, more than a helpful thing. You can sense from the friends that you know well enough where that would be appropriate and where it wouldn't be appropriate, and because I don't want to make light of it, I don't recommend it to just anybody who might see it as something harmful or wrong to do.

In other words, it's not something for everyone, if they have strong feelings against it, it probably wouldn't be good for them.

No, no, that's right. I think it certainly has to be someone who really feels that that's what they want to do. I don't think any of the women who are making that choice are doing it in ignorance or on a whim or because they think it's the thing to do, without a lot of personal reflection and consideration and study.

As you mentioned before, it was the mothering aspect of Darlene that stayed with you.

Yes, I really felt that as time went on I was relating to her almost as to a mother, someone who was looking after me as a mother would look after her own daughter, and that she had the kind of wisdom that comes from experience. That wisdom certainly ran deep.

Anna Fullerton

Anna (Toews) Fullerton was born in 1938 in Greenland, Manitoba, at home with a midwife. She and her husband, Bud, from whom she is divorced, have three children. Anna is a special education teacher and has lived in the Manitoba communities of Swan River, Brandon, Winnipeg, and Thompson. I interviewed her in Winnipeg.

Anna was introduced to me by Babs Friesen of the Women's Resource Centre at the YWCA, who knew I was interested in finding a midwife who had been active in the thirties and forties. Anna and I met and went together to visit the midwife who had assisted at Anna's birth, now living in a nursing home. Unfortunately, despite several attempts, she was too ill to undertake an interview. It occurred to me that Anna's story was as interesting as the midwife's, so we made two tapes together. I did not see myself as an interviewer with Anna, but as a midwife who sat with her in the spring twilight as she shared her look back at her childhood in a Holdeman home, and her childbearing years. Anna spoke with feeling of how her father was shunned within the Holdeman community.

I WAS BORN THE FIFTH CHILD in a family of ten. I went to Teachers' College, which was really not that common for women where I was from. Only a handful of women from the families there have gone into teaching.

I left my Holdeman roots at a fairly early age. I decided that it was too restrictive. There were so many things that I wanted to do and see, I just couldn't see myself staying in a narrow outlook like that. It was very hard at first, because I was ostracized. Only one of my brothers out of the ten children belongs to the church that my mother belongs to. But many of my brothers and sisters had never joined the church in the first place; I did. So when you leave or you are asked to leave, you have a stigma attached to you. I *wasn't* asked to leave, but they still made it very hard for me. As if I was really doing something very wrong. But I've certainly never regretted that. Because it's not me.

My father was a little more liberal-minded than many other people in the community, and then he was put out of the church. We were never told why, but his theories and his philosophy on life had a big bearing on the way I felt. I joined, I think more because the others my age were joining the church, and I wanted to belong. I think that was age twelve. There was a lot of pressure put on you to stand up, when they had the revival meetings. It's very difficult to be able to resist that pressure. It's such an alien sort of a world that people just don't understand.

And then to leave when I was so young — my mother of course didn't want me to leave, so I had the resistance from *her*. And sometimes, this was when I was in my teens, I would say things to her that she didn't agree with, she was really very angry with me, and a few times she would slap my face, and that just made me more angry than ever, of course. My father died when I was eighteen, when I was in Steinbach Collegiate. Before he died, I had written some of the ministers in the Greenland church to say that I did not want to belong to that church.

When my older sister and I joined the church, my father was already either put out of the church or he was leaning that way. He did not really encourage us to join. And when they had the first communion, which is a very grim, sobering experience in that church, with a lot of weeping and so on, foot washing also, he just would not let us go, and I was annoyed with him about that, but later I was so thankful that he had not allowed us to go to the first communion. And I never went. I sometimes felt that I would have liked to go out of curiosity, you can just imagine some of the atmosphere there. I used to go to members' meetings, where there was a very solemn, kind of grim atmosphere. I didn't really want anything like that.

What was discussed at these members' meetings?

Some of the things the people were not supposed to do, and people would sometimes stand up and confess their wrongdoings. I did that once. I can laugh about it now, but at the time and for years and years I felt very ashamed and guilty. Ashamed, more than anything, because I stood up in church and said that I was sorry that I had been wearing jeans to school. Now that sounds very trivial, but in those days you didn't do that in most communities, girls wore dresses all the time.

I wasn't very sorry for what I did. But I was under pressure to be like everyone else, to confess my wrongdoings. So it was more being made a public spectacle, that people will remember, and I felt dumb, kind of silly about it. For years I couldn't even talk about it. I never talked about it with my mother. Because she wasn't at that meeting. My sister was there. We just didn't talk about those things with my mother — in most ways she was against me. She was always on her church's side, and because she was under pressure to stay true to her traditions. She still is a member of the church. She is more understanding now of most of us, and she needs to be true to her traditions and we can accept that. But when you're an adolescent and you're rebelling and you're wanting to be independent, you're not going to be very sympathetic towards your mother.

I knew what I was up against, because of what they had done to my father, how hurt he was.There's a verse in the Bible, I used to know, but I don't really read the Bible any more, it says that you're to stay away from people who are dishonest, who lie, and — I can't even remember. To me it really means some fairly criminal activity, but people in the Holdeman church took this literally. Or they took it for the meaning they wanted to take. Because I guess people had this need for control, power, and if people who belonged to the church committed certain small misdeeds or misdemeanours, they would blow it up. They called it practising avoidance. My father had had a store in the community for many years. He wasn't really a farmer, he was happier in the store, and he was very friendly, he liked dealing with the public. He had more to do with other ethnic groups around us, he had many friends. But once he was not in the church any more, most [church] people would stop buying groceries. So of course that hurt the whole family, not just my father. Now tell me if that is Christian charity. That was deliberately done to hurt, not just my father, but the whole family. And then there's the avoidance when people of the church don't eat with the person who is involved. Now *that* I would say hurts. The other practice, for instance, when my father lost business at the store, that was economic, but this was deeper.

So members of his family who belonged to the church were not supposed to eat with him?

That's right, and really my mother wasn't supposed to either, but they weren't as strict then as they were a number of years later. So my mother continued to eat with my father. As far as I remember she did. And he almost stopped going to church, so she did too, she didn't go by herself. I think it was because she felt she had to go along with her husband, even though she had her own opinions, that was her place. I remember going to visit my father's brothers, and they would have my mother and father sit at the table first to eat, while they would sit and visit. That's not very comfortable.

When I saw these things happen it reinforced all those feelings of shame that I was talking about before, that we were always different, we were below, we were down on the ladder, but not just poor, we were different because of our religious beliefs. We were treated like second-class citizens, and that hurt. Really hurt, a very deep hurt. I don't know if you can ever really overcome that. You think you do, but I think it's always there. [pause] And then when I left the church, it was much different for me, because I wasn't at home that much, and I knew that it wouldn't affect me the same way as it had affected my father. But it still hurt. For years I refused to go back to the church in Greenland because of the way you were treated. You were either ignored, or people would say, "Oh, it's so good to see you back in church!" A few days before I got married, one of my friends that I used to go to school with came and visited and brought a gift and said, "Well, maybe you and your husband will both join the church." And I was angry, I was just furious. What right have you to say that to me? And it's so unrealistic, because nothing would ever be farther from the truth. I was very angry. But I still had that same feeling, that I didn't measure up, the same feelings of worthlessness.

Church somehow became something that came between family members.
Very much. Then there was that wave of persecution, I think it was in the early seventies. And there was a gulf that widened between some of our family members. After that my mother did not eat with me any more at the same table. Until perhaps the mid-seventies, she used to, but not any more. It doesn't bother me as much as it did for a while. My children don't like it, that's one reason they don't want to come to Grandma. I tried to explain it to them, but they couldn't understand.

Women have suffered very much in a church climate like that. Because women are not supposed to speak up at all. If anyone questions, it's the males. And the males are really the active ones. The women are just supposed to be quiet and go along and be good mothers, good wives, and do certain community work that just the women do, and it's the males that have the power. And God is seen as a male. So it's all very male-dominated. I never really heard about a God of love until I went to some other church meetings, I'd say the United Church more so. It was incredible.

I joined a Baptist church in Winnipeg, but later I found out that it was outwardly different from the one I had been a member of, but many things were the same, so I eventually left. After that I did not join any more churches. When I was married I went to a church that was evangelical also, but there was very little Christian charity there, I felt, when you really needed it, and that turned me off organized churches. That was it. I don't really consider myself a Christian now, I consider myself more of a humanist, I believe in the whole person.

Do you find some sense of community with other women?
Oh yes, I guess the first group of women that I really felt good about was when I went to work after I had left my marriage. It wasn't a professional type of work, but as it turned out, it really helped me in my healing. We used to have fun, there were three of us who were separated, and we all had children. I have had other groups since.

When you first found out you were pregnant, were you happy?
I was very happy. I had taught for three years in Swan Valley, and I had decided to stop teaching. At that time not many women worked after they were married, it wasn't really the custom then. We were on the farm and there was a lot of work. It was a new community for me, so that was a little difficult, but we lived near my husband's parents and some of his brothers, and I enjoyed being on the farm. But it was also a letdown, because I had been working for so many years and it was a very different life. But I was very happy to be pregnant. When I menstruated, I had a lot of problems, and I had been hoping that when I got pregnant and had a baby these difficulties would be overcome, and as it turned out, that's what happened. And with the first pregnancy I was really very anxious at times because my mother was not there. I talked with my sisters-in-law and asked them a lot of questions. There were no prenatal classes, but I felt fairly good through the first pregnancy.

Sometimes the doctor made me more anxious than ever. I had some pain in my tailbone, [laughs] and once he said, "You know, I might have to break your tailbone." Oh, that did not go over well. I think what he meant was during the delivery. I found out later that that was his way, he would talk before he thought many times. He wasn't thinking of his patients. In many ways, I felt fairly comfortable with him, but when the time came for the delivery, I was anxious.

I'll never forget that morning, May 20th, 1965. My water broke, very early, about five or 5:30 in the morning. It was a beautiful spring day. We drove to Benito. The birds were singing, it was such a lovely spring day, the sun was out. We came to the hospital and one of the nurses was very good to me. She also was there when I had the second baby. When I had such bad back pains, she would come and talk with me and hold my hand, and I appreciated that so much. Later I would talk about it, and people seemed to think that there was something the matter with me, that I needed that, as if I was talking too much about my emotions. I thought it was very normal for a woman to need another woman close by to comfort her and talk with her and hold her hand and rub her back.

It was a small hospital, a little nursing unit. I think I started to go into labour shortly after I got there, and the doctor told my husband to go have a cup of coffee and not to come back, because the baby probably wouldn't be born for hours. But as it turned out, the baby was born about two in the afternoon, so that my husband came back quite a bit later, and the baby was already born. He was surprised, I was happy that it was all over. The baby was a few weeks early, he was very long and kind of skinny, [laughs] he had some red marks on him, which worried me for a while, I think his nose was even folded over a bit. But the marks disappeared eventually.

And after the baby was born, well, who can describe the feeling of birth. The miracle of birth is always there, I think, after every birth. But the first baby, the first delivery, is always special because of it being the first. You've never had a child before that is part of you and part of your husband. It's something you can't really describe. It's just overwhelming, really, for a while. I think most women would feel that way, that it's very emotional. That here is something that's part of you, and before you were alone, then you got married, there were two, and now there are three! And then of course you realize the tremendous responsibility, that really hits you, too: I am responsible for rearing this child, and it's so new to you, it's frightening.

I'd like to go back to your not feeling good about leaving teaching, or your change in role. What was the part that you missed most about teaching?
My independence, definitely, my own paycheque. I had had my own car, and I had to get rid of it. I missed going places when I could go by myself, and I knew I would miss it, but I didn't realize how much. I used to go away for weekends, and then I'd have Christmas holiday, Easter holiday and summertime. I was bound now, and that was difficult. Also the teachers I worked with, or the people I met while teaching, they were in a different category, they were more professional than people I got to know after I was married.

And this was in a different place, so you didn't have any contact with those teachers any more?
Very little. I did have some contact at first with some of them, and one of them also married a farmer, but she didn't stop teaching. It was much later,

actually, that I realized how much I missed being with other people on a daily basis. It was a type of deprivation. But at the time you felt that you were doing what you were supposed to do, and you did it.

You wanted the children, but not at the expense of your independence?
Yes, in a sense I wanted to be at home, I wanted to have roots. I felt good about being on the farm and having roots and feeling like a part of the community, although that takes some time when you're going into a new community, especially if you're then raising children. But later I got to feel like a part of the community.

Could you talk a bit more about your first birth?
The birth itself wasn't really very long and I did not have a lot of problems. I did have some tearing, so I had to have stitches, I think about ten, and the nurses, the LPNs, they were very good, they talked with me during labour, and it was a very new experience for me. But it's something every pregnant woman knows she has to go through with, there's no way out, after nine months or shortly before, you know you have to go through with it. And that in itself sometimes causes a lot of anxiety. Some women have perhaps frightened you, because they've told horror stories, and you didn't really want to hear that, especially with the first pregnancy, so you try not to think about those things. And this was a small nursing unit. I had faith in my doctor, but this was my first baby!

I was breast-feeding the baby, and again, I had some anxiety; would I succeed, because I had really wanted to breast-feed, there was no comparison. And that was in the days when it wasn't really accepted. But my baby managed to eat fairly well. And then I had problems with sore nipples. Oh, I don't think I'll ever forget that. That was painful. And another thing that I won't forget is, when I was in the hospital, a few days after the baby was born, I had to have X-rays. And I remember how sore my breasts were, how *sore*, and how full. And not just that, but when I went for the X-ray, my nipples were dripping, constantly dripping away, and it was a little embarrassing and very painful and uncomfortable.

My mother came to stay with me about a week after he was born. I woke up that morning at five o'clock, I wanted the house cleaned up, and yet I wasn't very relaxed with the baby yet, because this baby was also causing me some trouble and loss of sleep. He was colicky, as I found out, and he cried a lot. Sometimes I didn't know what to do with him. When my mother came, we sat and chatted and I was still fairly tense, and then in the afternoon suddenly my milk was gone. I couldn't understand it, because I'd had so much milk. And here I didn't have any, what was the matter! My mother suggested that I was too tired, so I did go and rest. I think we probably gave the baby some juice, or whatever, and my mother probably rocked him to sleep, and I had a rest. Later the milk did come back, and I was very relieved. That never happened with the other children, because I learned that I had to have my rest.

How soon was your second child born?
A little less than two years after. Again, I had planned this baby. I was very anxious to have another one soon, because I felt that two children together, close in age, would be good. I knew it would be tough; I didn't know how tough. I had been on the pill some time after the first child was born, and also I found out, to my great relief, that my premenstrual troubles were over after the first baby was born. That was a terrific relief, because I used to get really sick, I used to get so sick I would hallucinate. And this didn't happen any more. But I was home, I wasn't working, and I felt I wanted a baby. With the second one I didn't get pregnant as soon as I wished, but that was really a blessing. I was fairly happy when I did, and yet, because I knew more of what was coming or what was supposed to come, I dreaded it a lot. But I also had timed it so that I would have the baby in the spring, because I felt that spring was the best time to have a baby, especially on the farm. Other women had talked about being pregnant in the hot hot summer, and I just couldn't face up to anything like that, so I had all my babies in the spring.

With my second baby I started having contractions very early, and it worried me. Then, I think it was in March, we had just had a very bad snowstorm, I was spotting, so I went to the doctor and he put me in the hospital. My sister-in-law was in the same hospital, she'd just had a boy, so I was in the same room with her, and I didn't want to be in the same room with her. I wasn't feeling that comfortable. But we did get to know each other a little better, and I did learn from her, it was her third baby. I ended up going home with no baby. It was false labour that I had. And the nurse said, "It's probably just as well that your baby has a little longer to mature, so he'll be healthier when he's born, or she." We wanted a girl, there were very few girls in the Fullerton family, in fact just one up to that point.

I was home for three more weeks when I started having pains, so I was back in the hospital at Benito, and again I didn't have the baby. I was getting a little impatient, but another storm came up, so I was very happy to be there. [laughs] My other boy was with Grandma and Grandpa, my husband's parents. I knew that he was in good hands. Well I thought he was; Grandpa sometimes told some colourful stories. [laughs] By that time my oldest was about two.

So one evening I realized the baby was going to come, and I believe it was two hours after the water broke. That was very short compared to the first one. The birth itself was not very eventful. This baby seemed to be a placid baby, and bigger than the first one. But then the afterbirth retained itself, and my doctor told me that I would have to have anesthesia and he would have to get hold of the nurse. This was at night, and the streets in the town were closed. So he phoned the nurse, and she came by skidoo. She gave me the anesthesia, and that was ether. I had never had ether before, and I've never since. I hope I never have it again, because I had some very strange experiences while I was under the drug. Later I realized that it was the ether that did it, but it was very strange. It felt like I was in a vacuum, in a time space, it was timeless, there was no time at all, and as if I had been there for centuries, and I was all alone. It was not a very good feeling. As I was coming to, I heard a ringing, and sometimes I hear those ringing sounds on the TV, and they remind me of that experience. I realized later that when I was starting to come out of the drug, that's when I had this, like a dream state. I heard the doctor and the devil, and the devil was bargaining with the doctor. The devil told the doctor: "I will let her go, if you admit that you made a mistake." I can't remember any of the details, but I just remember the awful experience of this part. I slowly woke up, and I could hear the doctor talking, and I could see him, and things began to be real again. I was out of that isolated timelessness, and gradually I forgot about that experience. I didn't talk to anyone about it until weeks later, I mentioned it to my younger sister, and she thought it was very interesting. Years later I asked my doctor because I thought I would really like to know, did he do something wrong during the surgery? He just laughed, he never said anything. Maybe he had done something, but he didn't want to talk about it. I wasn't supposed to know about it. Because the patient isn't supposed to know. I will never really know. Much later I realized it was all tied up with my feelings years before when I had left the Holdeman church, and how I was in Hades for three days. For three days after these ministers had met with me I felt that I was doomed eternally. And I'm sure my experience under ether was a subconscious replay of those earlier feelings. Some people would say, "That's nothing, it's just a dream."

But the baby was a happier baby, much more relaxed, I felt very close to the baby, and I breast-fed my second child for six months. And I guess being home more too, with the second one, and having the other child, we didn't socialize as much, so this second baby grew up to be much more quiet than the other children. I don't know if that had anything to do with it, it was his personality I think more than anything.

There were four years between my second and third child. I had planned it that way because I wanted a break. With the second pregnancy I was very depressed at times, extremely depressed, and in January or early February I wondered, how can I go through this, the months and weeks seemed so long and it was wintertime. At that time my husband got sick and had to stay in the house for two weeks. He started watching "The Edge of Night," a soap opera, and after he started, I got hooked on it, too. Also during my third pregnancy, I realized more than ever that there was something drastically wrong with our marriage. There were things that happened that I won't talk about now, but I was very lonely and depressed many times during the third pregnancy. I had to lie down every afternoon, because my varicose veins were very bad, and so I read a lot. I remember reading *The Grapes of Wrath.* Somebody told me not to, and I did get very depressed reading that book. I probably shouldn't have read it then, but I did, and somehow I got through that pregnancy.

Our daughter was born April 13th, 1971. For weeks before, I had to sit in a high chair, because I found it so hard to get up and sit down. And I was wearing my thick stockings, they weren't very pretty, [laughs] and of course there's a lot of work involved with two other children. Then again I was in the hospital early, but this time it was in Swan River, a bigger hospital, better equipped. My doctor had moved to Swan River by this time. But for me it was good, as I would find out later. I was put into the labour room when I got there, because I had labour pains, but then they stopped, and I was getting so bored. I was told to walk around. I felt conspicuous, but I did walk a fair bit. Then I had one of my attacks. For years I had had attacks of tachycardia, my heart would beat too fast. The doctor said it was nothing serious, but it scared me. I had one of those in the hospital, I had oxygen, but I felt, What if something happens to the baby? But nobody seemed very concerned about it. The third day I was in, I was so bored. My two boys were at Grandma's, and I knew that they were lonely, especially the younger one, so I thought I would go home the next morning, and just wait it out at home. But she was born that night, and I was in labour for about an hour. So that was very fast. She was a lovely baby, nine pounds two ounces, very nice looking, chubby baby.

But then things started to go wrong. Again, the doctor told me that I had the same thing, placenta retention, that I had had with the second baby, but this time I started hemorrhaging, and it was very scary, I'd never before had anything like that happen. After a while I could feel the life go out of me, starting at the tips of my toes. I wasn't scared, it was a very peaceful feeling, but I had just had a baby, I had had a girl, I had two children at home, I didn't want to die! I wasn't ready to die. The doctor was waiting for the other doctor, the anesthetist, who was busy sewing up someone's head wound downstairs, and I thought he would never get there, I thought I would die before he got there. And nobody seemed to be in any big panic. Later on I really was — annoyed isn't the word, I was furious about that, how I could have gone just like that, and they had not prepared for an emergency! The nurse who was on duty, the RN, was a very warmhearted, compassionate woman, and she helped me through this ordeal. I did not have ether this time, it was sodium pentathol, so I did not have the same unpleasant effects as with the second delivery. Finally the doctor came to administer the anesthesia, and when I saw his face, I was so happy, I was so relieved, and then before I knew it, I was under. And when I awoke I was told I was lying in a pool of blood, my bra was soaked, I just said throw it away. But I was alive. This was about five in the morning, and here I could have been dead, and I was not. I was alive. And that was a good feeling. I mean, that's the understatement of the day, but I survived. Phone my husband, I said. I knew he would be happy to have a girl, but I wanted him to realize, get him out of sleep and have him realize that I had nearly died, but I don't know if he ever really understood.

He was never with you with any of the births.
He was never there. He didn't want to particularly, and I guess maybe after a while I didn't either, because I felt that I could do it better on my own. And I think I was right. It wasn't really done then, either.

Did you have somebody help you at home?
Yes, but I found that fairly stressful, too. My husband was not very concerned about me, I think that hurt more than anything. This girl who came to help me, I had taught her at school, and I got along with her, she was good with the children, but there were things I had to teach her and I found that stressful. After she was gone, I had been at home for about six weeks, I started hemorrhaging. My husband wasn't home, and I was scared, really scared. So I phoned the doctor right away, and he said I should lie down immediately. And when I could get to the doctor, he put me back on birth control pills, and he said, "Your milk will slowly dry up," but it dried up much sooner than I thought it would, and I was very disappointed. But the baby was doing very well. Sometimes, though, she would throw up, it was like a geyser. I remember one night especially, I would be so tired. I would get up in the night and put her in bed with me and give her a bottle, and then just like that she would throw it all up, it would just gush out. I was concerned about that, but she was all right. She was a very healthy baby.

As for support from the family, some of my sisters-in-law were concerned, especially one of them. We got together a lot, we were fairly close for a long time. There were two other women in the district who also had a baby about the same time. I would get together with other women. And now two of these girls are very close, my daughter and one of them.

What about your relationship with your mother? You mentioned it improved after you had children.
Oh, yes. After I had the first baby I felt very close to her, because now I had what I was supposed to have, I was married, I was on a farm, I had a child, and I was at least the closest to what she wanted of me! Yes. And she did give me a fair amount of advice about babies.

Is there anything you would have done differently?
Perhaps yes, but at the time I couldn't, because I had my mind made up about certain things. Later on, when I found it hard having to discipline the children mostly on my own, take care of them on my own, I often thought that I should never have had children, I wasn't really a fit mother. I wasn't patient enough, I needed more room for myself.

On the other hand, did you have an example of your mother taking time for herself? Can one have children and also have a life of one's own?
Well, my mother did in her way, she had her retreat by reading. She used to read and my oldest sister would be like a second mother to us. Or we would take care of ourselves, which we did a lot. So yes, my mother did, if you want to call it that, have time for herself. But there were so many things where there was no comparison between when I raised my children and when she raised hers, things were so different.

Certainly now I'm very happy that I had my three children. Now one of them tells me that he will never have children. But I also know that he may change his mind. Nowadays there isn't the pressure to raise children, your own or anyone else's. And I probably wasn't ready to have children, but then, would I ever have been?

Robyn Epp

Robyn (Warkentin) Epp was born in 1964 in Winnipeg. She is a music teacher who has lived in the Manitoba communities of Meadows, Boissevain, and Leaf Rapids. She and her husband, Ernie, have two children. Robyn's own birth is described by her mother, Agatha Warkentin, elsewhere in this book.

With the warmer spring weather I headed out to Boissevain, about 288 kilometres from Winnipeg, where I interviewed three women: twenty-four-year-old Robyn, who had her first baby at age twenty; Gertrude Epp (Robyn's husband's grandmother), a woman in her eighties; and my sister Elsa, who was in her fifties. I have known Robyn since she was a little girl. She is diabetic, and the stories of her pregnancies are dramatic, with their details of the close medical supervision required by her condition.

I WAS VERY EXCITED TO FIND OUT that I was pregnant with Marli, who is four now, and everyone else was excited, too. With me being diabetic, I set off on a nine-month course of hard work, because to have a healthy pregnancy and a healthy baby, you have to really strive for normal blood sugars and keeping the diabetes under control. I found that a real challenge. I ate exactly what I was supposed to, I didn't even have a chocolate chip cookie! I did glucose monitoring every day, for the next seven, eight months.

I find it hard to remember exactly how that pregnancy went, except for the times that I had to go into the hospital, twice, once right after

Christmas, because at that point my blood sugars were too high, I guess the hormones produced by the pregnancy were fighting against the effects of the insulin, and that made it go out of control, regardless of what I did. I found that frustrating, I was really concerned that everything would go well. I went into the hospital for a week then, that was over 1983 into '84, and when I got out my husband and I moved to Winnipeg for three months, because I had fetal assessment twice a week. We lived in my grandparents' house, we were housesitting for them, and my husband got a job in the bank where he had worked before we'd moved here, so he had something to do. And then on February 7th, I went into the hospital, and I stayed in for a whole month till the baby was born on March 6th. At first I thought, I'll just be in for another week, and then it kept stretching, and finally it clicked in that I was going to be there till the baby was born! I found that hard, because I was cooped up. I did a lot of needlework and read. Ernie came to visit, and I didn't even get to go home on weekends until the weekend before the baby was born. Then they let me out for two days. I was well rested, I wasn't tired, I could sleep when I wanted, didn't have to do any housework, but emotionally that was hard, I was really alienated from people around me. I was in the women's hospital, and there were all these other women there with high blood pressure or whatever. But I had these roommates that kept coming in for two days and then leaving. I was there for five weeks and these people were there for a few days. I can't even remember how many people shared that room with me. There had to be at least six. I was patiently waiting, and waiting and waiting, I never really expected that I would go into labour or anything.

What do you mean, you didn't expect to go into labour?

I didn't think I would go into labour. It would be: Oh I want this baby to be born! and the doctors would come in and say: "Well, just hold on a little longer." They brought me up to thirty-nine weeks, and they really watched closely. I had an amniocentesis at about thirty-six weeks, and they said no, the baby wasn't ready. My diabetes wasn't affecting it that badly yet. One doctor said to me he was concerned that the placenta would give out because of the sugars, which I guess is possible, so they watched me closely. They did another amniocentesis, and they said the baby was ready. So they said, "We'll try inducing." The next day they took me to the labour ward at 6:30 in the morning, and they started applying a prostaglandin suppository, to ripen my cervix, to get it ready. I started having mild contractions that lasted all day. And then for some reason they stopped doing it, I guess they didn't want me to go into labour. I look back now and I think, Why didn't they just let me try it? But they stopped it, for whatever reason. They left it and said, "We'll try again on Monday."

So they let me out for the weekend. I had a great time with Ernie. We went to this carnival at Meadows, I was walking around big as a house it seemed like, and then the next day we went to some friends' and had a nice "this is it" party, and on Monday I was in the labour ward again, and they started me on the I.V. drip, and that I found really hard. I had three heparin locks in, in three different places. One for the I.V., one was for the hormone to start labour, Oxytocin I guess, and then they had a heparin lock in because they were testing my blood sugars every two hours. I look back at that now and I think, oh that was just awful. I was really hooked up. I had a fetal monitor on me, I had things going. And I just lay there, and I felt like I wasn't even important. The nurse would walk in for the next shift and say, "Well, how's the machine doing?" They wouldn't ask how *I* was doing. I felt like this was just one big experiment. You know? And nothing happened. I didn't have any contractions, just mild little things, nothing big. Obviously I wasn't ready to go into labour.

I was there from 6:30 in the morning, and finally about six that night they said, "OK, nothing's happening, we'll unhook her and try again tomorrow." I was so disappointed. I went to the phone and called Mom, and I cried, I said, "Nothing happened." I had to go through that again tomorrow. I had fully thought, Well if nothing happens all day, they'll do a Caesarean. Today! But they said, "No, we'll try it tomorrow." So next morning again at 6:30 they hooked me all up again. I went through the whole thing again. They tested my blood sugar, one through my finger every hour, and every two hours they did one that they would get through a vein. And because they put the heparin in they had to take it out of the lock, so that it wouldn't contaminate the blood, so they were taking two big things of blood out of me every two hours. I was getting really weak, I was shaking on the table. And finally my obstetrician came in and said, "You know, nothing's happening." He did a vaginal, and he said, "You're not even dilating. We may as well do a Caesarean." By that point, I was so happy, I was ready to jump on the table and say, "Hallelujah!" [laughs] That was about 3:30 in the afternoon. I said, "Great, let's go for it," because I'd been hooked up for two days, and it was terrible.

Maybe if I had been older I would have objected more, or questioned more what they were doing, but I just said, "OK, we'll do this," because they were the doctors. So I had an epidural, and we'd made sure that Ernie could be there to experience it, the doctor really believed in it. I've talked to a lot of my girlfriends about that, and none of them had had their husbands in at all.

Having the Caesarean was really rather interesting. It was a little nauseating, they had it hooked so I could see what they were doing. I watched as they cut and then I couldn't watch any more, it was too red, too much blood. But I could see when she was born, and then I cried, because I was so excited. It took forty-five minutes, approximately. I felt so relieved, but I was shaking, because I was very anemic. I didn't have enough blood, very low iron, so I had a hard time recovering from that. I was so tired emotionally and physically from what I'd gone through for two days. I was really up for when she was born, but I remember later, lying in the recovery room, I felt like I was paralyzed, I was cold and shivering, and I could hardly move; they were trying to get me to move my legs, because it helps to recover faster. That was really hard.

The next couple of days are actually kind of a blur. It was kind of a hazy pain, and because I was so anemic, I was weak, so when they tried to get me up the first time, I felt like I was collapsing, and finally I guess they realized that I was anemic, because I had two blood transfusions. That made me feel better. In fact Mom said, "You looked so gray, and when you were getting that blood, you could just see the colour coming back." I had a hard time recovering the next few days. I don't know whether it was just that I didn't know what to expect from a Caesarean, and the pain, or maybe all the confusion and the exhaustion that I had gone through.

It's hard to know which things are due to what, because you've never experienced it before.
That's right. The second time it was different, because I knew exactly what to expect, and I prepared myself for it. It took a little convincing for me, actually, to have a second one, because I kept remembering, and I was certainly glad it wasn't too soon after having Marli that I got pregnant. I think I would have been devastated if it had happened even in the first year. It took quite a while for me emotionally to recover from that. And I don't know if I'm still — I have a hard time talking about it, because of the feelings — and the thing is, I'm so happy, I'm happy that I have a child, but I have such mixed feelings about the birth, because of everything that I went through, and I really trusted my doctors, but there were other ones that I felt so — I was used. When I went on the labour ward that first time, they were doing some things that — I just felt they were so rude to your person. I lost all sense of modesty there — I don't know, how graphic do you want me to get?

You can say anything you want. It's up to you.
OK, OK. Well it was just, I really felt they were inconsiderate of women. I was a nineteen-year-old girl, and — I don't know how they are with normal deliveries — I realized I was a high-risk pregnancy, but a lot of them weren't

concerned about how I was feeling, it was just, let's get this baby born, it was like the body and the diabetes were so much more important. Some of these residents — there was this one man, he sticks out in my mind. He did a vaginal check, and he didn't use lubricant! He was really rough. My obstetrician came in, and the nurse handed him just this disinfectant, and he said, "Where's the lubricant?! I can't do this without lubricant!" and I thought, no wonder that other thing hurt so bad! I felt like I was just being pressed against the wall, and it hurt so bad, because I'd only had one before, they just never did them routinely. My mom said she had them routinely, well I didn't, because they were doing fetal assessment, that sort of thing, and this guy was so inconsiderate! So I lost a lot of sense of modesty after that, because I felt, they don't care, so I shouldn't feel embarrassed. I never was embarrassed, I always felt I had a pretty open mind to that, but that really bothered me that that happened, it was so unfair. And inconsiderate.

I felt like an experiment, and after, too, when they were experimenting with my blood sugars. I wasn't quite sure what they should be doing with my insulin after the baby was born, like there was a drop and the whole bit. I must have started off taking about forty units of insulin, a split dose. By the time I was at thirty-nine weeks, I had to take two needles in the morning, because there was too much for the syringe. That was hard, that sense of being out-of-control, because when you're diabetic you're always wanting to be *in* control. So after Marli was born, my diabetes doctor was away, and when he came back I asked about my diet. I wasn't sure if I was getting a diabetic soft diet, because I was eating puddings and things that were so sweet, I thought, I don't think they even know I'm diabetic! I was really confused and concerned. When he heard that, he went to the nurses' desk and said, "What the hell's going on here, what are you doing with my patient!" They were experimenting! It was like — let's try this! Let's try that!

Even the term "high risk" set me back the first time I heard it. It must have been about the first week with the first pregnancy at fetal assessment, somebody said "high risk," and I thought, Oh, I guess I am! I hadn't thought of myself in those terms at all! And so that took me back, and even that, you can have the feeling, like, hooo! I feel like a guinea pig! They look at you as if you're something really different. I guess their primary concern is that you have a healthy baby, but a lot of the medical stuff sure gets in the way of that. They're more concerned about how the machines are working than how you're feeling, like just that experience of being induced. That was so degrading! you know? This one nurse actually walked in and said, "Well, how's it doing? How's it doing?" *It*. Not, how is *she*, how are *you*, it was how is *it*. I felt like I was plugged into a machine. And that was a very terrible feeling. About four o'clock in the afternoon this person walked in and I felt like saying forget it! and ripping everything off. I said, "I'm doing fine." I figured, you know, I'm supposed to have a baby here, [laughs] not be the medical experiment. I don't know if it's possible for a diabetic to have a birth without all that paraphernalia around. It was a little easier the second time.

How did you feel about breast-feeding?
I wanted to breast-feed. And I had a hard time with Marli, for some reason. She wouldn't latch on right, so — this is going to sound crazy, but I used a nipple from a bottle and I put it over my nipple, and she could get it through that, but she wasn't getting a lot. But I remember I was so frustrated trying to get her to nurse and she wouldn't, and then the nurse would come in and say, "Here!" and then she'd grab her head and kind of cram her face against me, they just wouldn't let me have enough time, and I kept thinking, I can hardly wait till I'm home, and I can do this on my own! You know? I was so fed up with being in the hospital, I'd been there for five weeks. I was ready to go home. It took a week to recover from the surgery. Then it took me a good month to get her to latch on properly. I was just determined that that's what I wanted to do. I'm basically lazy, I didn't want to have to sterilize bottles. [laughs] It was easier just to breast-feed, and I really enjoyed it. It takes a while to recover from a Caesarean, and I was also anemic. We stayed at Mom and Dad's for another three weeks, where I really had it easy, I didn't have to come home and cope all by myself.

We moved home at the end of March, and I had a great summer, I enjoyed having a baby. And it was worth it, too, all that hard work for the nine months before, I really enjoyed her. I've had a few more struggles with her now growing up, [laughs] but I guess trying to balance everything that I'm trying to do, or want to do, plus having them, makes it harder.

How did your second pregnancy and birth compare with the first?
With Jonathan, we had planned when we were going to have him, so we were very careful that we didn't have an "accident," because I knew I'd have to go to Winnipeg for two months beforehand to have fetal assessment, and that meant moving in with my parents. I wanted to plan it for a time when it would suit them, too, as well as myself, because I was teaching in my home by that time, so I wanted to have a good year of teaching. It was a half-year, as it turned out. I was very excited at first, with him, plus I was leery, kind of dreading having to go through it again. Ernie was more excited than I was, he wanted a second child more than I did at that point. So again I started nine months of really watching, monitoring my blood sugars and everything, and I felt really good. I got a lot of rest, because Marli was still

having a nap at that point, I could lie down with her, and I did a lot of that.

The first time I went to my obstetrician, I was really leery about being induced again, so I asked him if I had to go through that, and he said, "Well quite frankly, you went through two days of hell last time, I don't think we'll make you go through that again." That put some of my fears away, because I knew I didn't have to face that. And if I went into labour, fine, but probably it would be planned Caesarean. I always thought I didn't really care how I gave birth, whether it was a vaginal or a Caesarean, I just wanted to have the baby. Because I'm working so hard to have a healthy baby, as long as she or he arrives, who cares how it happens. I would read these books about giving birth, and how some women are so geared up for natural childbirth, and then if they have a Caesarean, they have such a sense of failure, and I never had that feeling at all. Having a Caesarean is a painful way of giving birth, because it's so medical. But if a healthy baby is the end result, it doesn't matter.

So anyway, because I kind of knew what would happen, I felt more at ease, and I managed to stay out of the hospital the whole time, that was really great. I moved to Mom and Dad's in the beginning of May, and twice a week Mom drove Marli and me to Winnipeg to Health Sciences, where I had fetal assessment. I got to know them really well there; I knew the receptionist, because she had worked at the Diabetic Education Centre. I got to know everyone else through her. So that was really great, I could come in and say, "Hi, how are you," and it was really a nice feeling.

I enjoyed fetal assessment, because it's so intriguing to see how your baby is growing and measuring the bones, and seeing these things; you could see that he had hair, once he got a little further along, and it was really neat, really fascinating. It takes ultrasound waves of the baby and then they have a computer keyboard there, and they can do a digital measurement of the bones and the head circumference and the abdomen, so they see the baby is growing at a healthy rate, and they can judge the birth weight, or the weight of the baby. He started off at about six pounds, then six and a half, seven, seven and a half. We kept thinking, Oh my goodness, this kid's getting bigger and bigger, and I was getting bigger. [laughs]

It was really hot that summer, and I didn't have any summer clothes, because I had been pregnant with Marli fall and winter, so I had to go out and buy clothes, and luckily I did it before that week, it was thirty degrees that week, I was so hot, oh! And that was only in May, and I was due middle of July, and I kept thinking, Oh, I don't know how I'm going to survive! We kept watching, and at one point I had a little bit more amniotic fluid than I should have, so they said, "You better stay off your feet a bit, because if this continues, you will be in the hospital." So that meant that

Mom did a lot of running after Marli, because she was two at that point, and very active. I'm very indebted to her and Dad. I came back home pregnant, and with a two-year-old, after I'd been married four years already, and they had to have the pressure of my ups and downs and missing my husband, because he was here in Boissevain, he came and saw us on weekends. That was hard on the marriage and hard on the family. We survived it, but we didn't think there would be a third one.

About three weeks before the due date my doctor said, "Well, I think we should book the delivery room for your Caesarean," and I was a little taken by surprise, I thought, Three weeks? I thought, Oh! OK. This must have been about the beginning of June, and I thought this was a bit early, but in three weeks, who knows. He was thirty-seven weeks when he was born.

"Normal" is about forty, is it?

Yes, but he was almost nine pounds then, so I was relieved. As it was, when they did the Caesarean, he made the incision a bit too small, he couldn't get a good grab on his head, so he had to use forceps to get him out, it was amazing! [laughs] I couldn't believe it! — They did an amniocentesis on the Wednesday, Ernie was still in Boissevain. He said, "Phone me as soon as you know." So finally they said, "Yes, the baby's lungs are mature, so we'll have the Caesarean on Friday morning." Even that was booked, because my diabetes doctor was away that week. He wasn't too crazy about it, he's like a mother hen when his diabetic patients have babies, he was so much support actually. If I had a problem, he would see me right away, and I was there a lot, he gave me a lot of support. So finally I found out, phoned Ernie, I think he made it in two hours [laughs] — it's a three-hour trip.

The next day I went into the hospital, Thursday afternoon. We were so much more positive the whole way! I tried to go to sleep that night, but I woke up at 5:30 in the morning, and it was a beautiful day. I just lay awake there, thinking, and I had a much more relaxed and peaceful feeling about it, you know. I knew that the baby was going to be born, and I knew I didn't have to go through what I'd gone through the time before. Ernie came at 6:30, he had hardly slept that night either, and we went to the labour floor, and I had another epidural, and I remember lying there joking with the anesthesiologist and the doctors. We were all so excited, because it wasn't an emergency. We weren't tired, we weren't emotionally tired, we were really up for everything, and so it was a really positive thing. I felt so upbeat about it, the relief of knowing that it wasn't going to be the same type of thing as the first time.

I look back at that first birth now, and I still can hardly talk about it without sounding bitter or hurt, because it did hurt, it hurt physically and mentally, to have that happen. The only thing is, I don't want Marli to have guilt, or bad feelings about it, because I was happy to have her. But I guess because of the diabetes you just don't know what it's going to be like till you're going through it. And I was pretty determined with the second to have it more positive, and not so much feeling confused or left out. I felt more informed and that attitude must have been picked up, because I felt much more at ease with everyone.

You were more in control of what was going to happen.
Yeah. Still the doctor called the shots about when the baby was going to be born. Three weeks before, he said, "We'll pick this day, because next week I'm going on my holiday." And I thought, Oh dear! So I went to my diabetes doctor, and he said, "I'm in L.A. that week, you can't have the baby then!" I said, "Well, my obstetrician can't be there, because the next week *he's* going away!" So that was funny! Because they couldn't get together. Anyway, my diabetes doctor came back and right away came to see me, and he was really excited that I'd had a healthy baby.

Do you think that somebody who knows a little more about diabetes and pregnancy and giving birth could have given you some help in preparing for the first one, or is there no way that you could be prepared?
I think it would have helped to read some case histories of what a diabetic's experience was. I remember reading once that a woman had had three Caesarean births and they were all fine, but it was in no detail. And I think if I had had something to read or someone tell me, "This was exactly what my experience was, it might be like this," it might have helped. I read a lot before, about birth in general and breast-feeding, to get prepared for that, and we went to the prenatal classes here in Boissevain. But that was all geared basically for vaginal birth and also for someone who would have a normal and not a high-risk pregnancy.

Do you feel that birth is more than just a physical experience, does it change you in any way, having children? The birth itself.
Yeah. It did change me, because it made me grow up. I was exposed to some things that I hadn't been exposed to before that changed me, you know. It made me feel that you shouldn't implicitly trust a doctor just because he's a doctor, because they don't always know best. Not the doctors I had. I have a very close relationship with the diabetes doctor, so I trust him. The obstetrician took a little longer, but I did trust him too, because he would listen to me, and he kind of understood how I felt. But these other ones that I just kind of met, they're not sensitive enough to people. — I can't say

objectively how it's changed me, I don't think. I haven't figured that out yet. Maybe it'll take me another twenty years to figure that one out. Sometimes I wonder now, why did I have kids?! I didn't expect raising children to be quite as difficult at times as it is; maybe that's what I'm thinking. I didn't look past having the baby stage. And the babies are easy compared to having the toddlers, I feel.

Elsa Neufeld

Elsa (Klassen) Neufeld, my sister, was born at home on the family farm near Halbstadt, Manitoba, in 1932. She and her husband, Werner, have three children. She has lived near Boissevain most of her life and now lives in Winnipeg. Elsa has taught driver education and has worked in personal care homes.

I stayed overnight with Elsa at her home. While I asked questions about her pregnancies and childbirth she sat and ripped open the seams of a discarded pair of jeans for patching material. It is always a surprise to me that, while I think I know my sisters well, there are many gaps in my knowledge of their lives. Elsa is a pragmatic, down-to-earth person, and she seems to have had her children in a like manner. In addition to the story of the births of her own children, she tells of the arrival of her grandson, Ezra, in a planned home birth at her residence in 1987.

I GREW UP IN A FAMILY of fifteen children. I was one of the middle children, and having taken care of my little brothers quite extensively, I wasn't in any hurry to start my family when I got married, in fact, my husband and I agreed that we would wait three years before we had a child. Of course, we didn't have any birth control, but we just weren't going to have any children. My older sister had waited five years before she had her first baby and she wasn't using any birth control, so I thought I would be the same way. I did ask my married sisters and one sister-in-law for birth control advice, and my sisters couldn't give me any birth control advice except one who said abstinence, and I said to her, "Well, your first baby wasn't born till you were married more than a year, and you must have used something," and she said no! The sister-in-law told me to use vinegar douche, immediately after intercourse, and that would ensure that I would not get pregnant. So I diligently vinegar-douched, but I got pregnant anyway. Got pregnant twice on the vinegar douches, actually.

I was married ten months when we had our first child. And I really enjoyed having Debbie, but the second child was born nineteen months later, so by the time we were married three years we had two children! And sometimes I thought that maybe they lacked some of my attention, because I had done so many activities with my little brothers that as far as I was concerned I had done them, and I didn't want to do them again. But our third child was born five years after the second one, so I think in terms of time spent with her, she suffered the most, because by that time I had done all these little projects with two sets of children, with my little brothers and with my first two children, so that I wasn't into doing some of those things, and also it just didn't seem worthwhile with just one child.

When you first found out you were pregnant, whom did you tell?
I don't recall telling anybody very quickly. My pregnancies were during the time when it was the thing to keep it secret as long as possible, and you tucked in your tummy when you were in public and tried to keep it secret for at least four months, and if you managed to keep it secret longer, so much the better. And so I can't really recall whom I told and how soon. Also one lady in the church had said to me, since my mother had had fifteen children, "Well I guess you're going to have fifteen children, too." And I was horrified, that was the last thing I wanted, and so I certainly was not going to let anybody know that I was pregnant, because I was not going to be labelled as having fifteen children.

My periods were somewhat irregular, so I never was really sure that I was pregnant until I was at least two months pregnant. And so I likely wouldn't have told anybody till about three months, and probably waited till about four months. And I remember the first pregnancy. We were killing chickens at Whitewater at Wern's parents' place, and not knowing the symptoms of pregnancy, I had mentioned to my sisters-in-law and my mother-in-law that I had a voracious appetite, that whenever I had a noon sleep I would wake up just famished. And I'm sure that they then realized that I was pregnant, but I didn't think about that, that I was giving myself away, but I remember on that chicken-killing day, which would have probably been October, that was when I told them that I was pregnant and they were quite surprised, because they had thought that I would be smarter than they were, and that I wouldn't be pregnant so quickly. This shock value seemed to be something that people enjoyed in those days, to shock people when you told them that you were pregnant.

Did you feel you got enough prenatal advice from your doctor?
I guess I was rather fortunate, I had a female doctor, and she was quite good at telling you things, for instance, she advised me to prepare my nipples ahead of time if I was going to nurse, and I thought that was very good advice. Yes, I think there were a lot of details that she helped us with that probably a male doctor, especially at that time, would not have thought of telling us.

Was there any restriction on activities?
I had very good health during my pregnancies, my in-laws always told me I glowed when I was pregnant, and I never had any morning sickness or any problems at all, with any of the pregnancies. The first pregnancy, I didn't realize how easily I would gain weight, and also since we had no refrigeration, and in those days you didn't buy fruit and vegetables like you do now, I filled up on carbohydrates, and I did gain a lot of weight. I had been ninety-eight pounds when I got married, and nine or ten months later I was 140-some pounds, so that was quite a difference.

Would you say you were confident, or how would you describe your feelings about pregnancy?
Confident and not knowing enough to really worry. I had not had much experience at all with handicaps or even seeing handicapped children, and so it never entered my mind to worry about birth defects or anything like that. Certainly there was some worry about the birth itself, especially towards the end, but I guess you sort of think, well, all these other women have made it, you'll make it, too.

Was your labour very long with Debbie?
I noticed my labour pains in the morning when we woke up, probably around seven or eight in the morning, and we went to the hospital around four o'clock in the afternoon, and the baby was born around 11:30 at night. So it was not really fast, but not that long either.

And no complications or anything?
No complications. Of course I had never been hospitalized before, so just being in a hospital was a new and kind of a frightening experience, because

you didn't know what was happening, and they wouldn't give me any supper that evening. I was very hungry and couldn't understand why they wouldn't give me any supper. Later on I knew why. The shaving was, I don't know, not a pleasant experience.

There were a lot of associations with being sick, probably.
Oh yes. Which I actually really enjoyed, being pampered, having my meals served, I enjoyed that part. I stayed at least a week, and didn't get out of bed for at least two or three days.

Was Wern interested in being with you in labour, and was he able to?
That wasn't even a consideration, it wasn't even talked about at that time. By the third time, by the time Vicki was born, then we were asking about it, and they said no. They said the labour room was too small, they didn't have room for fainting husbands in there.

What about the staff, was it a fairly small hospital?
Yes, a small hospital. OK, the first two births I was well taken care of. By the third birth, I had taken some prenatal care, and I had learned some breathing techniques, and so I felt more confident, but I was unfortunate to have a very unsympathetic nurse. I said to her, "I feel like bearing down," and she said, "It's much too soon!" When I rang the bell the second time and said, "I feel like bearing down," she got very angry with me and she said, "OK, we'll have to get you out of this room if you're going to make such a fuss." She was very short with me, very abrupt, and she made me get up out of bed and walk to the delivery room, she made me climb onto the delivery table, which — none of it really hurt me, but I knew I wasn't to be treated like this. Meanwhile my husband phoned to ask when this baby was going to be born, this was around eight o'clock in the morning, and she told him, "Oh, this baby won't be born till about noon." She was just barely off duty when my baby was born.

Is there anything that stands out? Can you tell me about David's birth?
David was born on December 15th. He was three weeks overdue. We didn't have a good road past our place, and we had very much snow that winter, so one evening when I was more than two weeks overdue, we had a very bad blizzard, and I phoned my doctor and said, "What if I have to come in tonight?" And she said, "Just pray that you won't have to. And tomorrow make sure you get into town and stay here until the baby is born." So the next day I went to town by horse and sleigh, and I stayed with friends of the family [Gertrude and Bernhard Epp]. She was fifty-eight and he was sixty,

and she began giving me advice, like that I should take a hot bath and that would bring on the baby, and I should take castor oil — I'm not sure whether I took castor oil, but I know I took the hot bath, I took a hot bath two nights in a row, and the third morning I started feeling labour pains early, maybe around five o'clock in the morning, and I did not want to wake up these old people, in case it was a false alarm, so I tiptoed down the stairs and sat and knitted and watched the clock there, but about fifteen or twenty minutes later the lady of the house was downstairs too, she had heard me, and we watched the clock together for a while, and then we decided to phone the doctor, and the doctor said, "Go to the hospital." So this sixty-year-old man went out to back out the car, and being somewhat excited, he got the car stuck in the driveway, and I volunteered to come and help push, but they said, "No no no no!" [laughs] So they took me to the hospital, and my husband was peacefully sleeping at home. The first thing I said to the delivery nurse was that I was really quite uptight because my husband was not able to take me in, and she said, "Well, that's no good," and she gave me an injection, which I'm sure was some kind of a tranquilizer, and I had a very easy birth. David was born within three hours, and it was so much easier than Debbie's had been.

The doctor always made it in time?

Yes. With my first baby, Debbie, it seemed like a very long labour because I was in hard labour for several hours, and my back was so sore. And I guess also because I was under anesthesia, I was telling my doctor all kinds of things, and one of the things I said to him was, "And my mother had fifteen! How did she ever do it!" And I said to him, "I'm never having another one!" [laughs] And when I left the hospital, he said, "See you next year!"— Previously I said I had a lady doctor, this was a husband and wife team, he did the delivery and she did the prenatal care. — I did have stitches with Debbie, and they opened and were very painful.

They opened immediately after, you mean?

Well actually they opened after I got home, because I was trying to clean up my house to impress my mother-in-law, and was doing too much. It was just dreadfully painful, I had to use a heat lamp and what not all to heal them.

You breast-fed all of your children, didn't you?

Oh, that's another story, yes. I was not affirmed in this at all in this community. The bottle had come in and we had been liberated and why would I even think about breast-feeding! But I persevered, and when we were visiting, I was isolated, I had to sit alone in a room, because it just wasn't done, to uncover yourself, even with good nursing bras or blankets over, it just wasn't done, you did not expose yourself, not even in front of other women. You sat alone in a room and you nursed your child. So at those times I would feel a little isolated, I would have rather been in the other room, chattering away, but I had to sit there by myself and feed this child.

How would they enforce that? Were remarks made if you did it, or didn't you even dare to do it?
You just wouldn't even think of doing it anywhere else, and you even felt self-conscious doing it in the cry room at church, where nobody could see anything. It was sort of — you just felt that people wondered why in the world you would do such a thing.

Did people really ask you too, or did you just hear about it?
No, no, some would say it right to you, they would ask, why are you doing that?

And why did you do it? Obviously most people weren't doing it, how did you come to the conviction that it was a good thing?
Well, I'm not sure. I know my one sister-in-law did, and I was impressed with it, and I knew that it was best for the child. And I'm sure that cost wasn't a consideration, because we milked our own cows, so it wasn't as if we'd be buying the milk. I did like the convenience of it, too.

Your doctor must have supported you in it, too.
Yes, she supported me. Yes, I think she was actually quite supportive of breast-feeding. But most of my contemporaries, the women who had babies at that time were not breast-feeding, there was probably one or two who did, but most of them were not.

In what ways was your church a support to you? Either with having children, or any other way.
Most of the people in church are baby lovers. So you always felt very special when you came to church with a new baby. Everybody wanted to see the baby and you just felt really special. And not only with a new baby, people were always interested in your child. Not only in church, but any time they met you. Children are considered special, and I think it's still that way.

So now you're a grandmother. What has that experience been like?
Well, our oldest daughter had rheumatoid arthritis and diabetes when she

was ten years old, and so I was not really anxious for her to start a family, I was concerned about her health. So I had said to her, you don't need to have a child just to make me a grandmother. And just before she got pregnant, she and her husband had been planning to quit their jobs and take a trip to Europe, and I thought that was a great idea. When I was told she was pregnant, I wasn't all that overjoyed, I was more in favour of the trip to Europe! But after the child was born, he was really special. Maybe I should go back to the day he was born. She was hospitalized early because of swelling in her feet and we weren't really expecting her to have the baby at that time because it was premature, but one morning Bob called and said that they thought the baby would be born that day, so we drove into Winnipeg and we thought we'd be there when this great event happened. And then nothing happened, and it was seeding time, this was in May, so we went back home, and two days later he phoned and said the baby would be born that day. I had to do something to keep myself busy, I didn't know what to do with myself, so I gave my bathroom one good cleaning, from corner to corner that day! And by the time my bathroom was spotless, I had a grandson in Winnipeg. Then I thought, Well, I'm not going to be one of these crazy grandmothers who's forever ranting and raving about my beautiful grandchild. We did go to Winnipeg to see our grandson, and he had been seven weeks premature, so he was in an incubator, and we didn't get to hold him the first time we saw him, and of course in an incubator you don't see as much of them, either. When I came back home, my sister-in-law asked me, "Well, how was the grandson?" and I thought, well, I was going to play it cool, so I just said, "Oh fine!" And she thought to herself, there must be something wrong with that baby! [laughs] Well I soon forgot about not being like the other grandmothers and I started bragging about my beautiful grandchildren just like everyone else.

So he was the only grandchild for quite a while.
Yes, he was. By that time our son and our younger daughter were married, and I had said to the older daughter, "I don't think you should have another baby," because her arthritis really flared up after Michael was born. Then we went to visit our son and his wife in Africa, and they were talking about having a baby, and I said I would feel absolutely gypped if I had a grandchild in Africa! So I had told them not to have one. Then I went home and I told my youngest daughter, you're so young, you have lots of time, don't be in a hurry to start your family! Well about a month later I heard that they were all three pregnant, they were all expecting in November!

So much for grandmotherly advice!
Yes.

I'd like to hear about the home birth in your family, if you want to describe that?

Oh! [laughs] OK! When our son and daughter-in-law came back from Africa with their two-year-old daughter Kholiswa, they were planning their second child, and meanwhile they had talked to some midwives, and although they were living in Saskatoon, they were impressed with a midwife near our place in Manitoba. So one day our son was talking to his father on the telephone and he was saying that it was too bad they couldn't have this midwife that lived near our place, and I was on another telephone and I heard my husband saying to our son, "Well I guess there's no reason why you can't have the baby here!" And I didn't say anything, but my son somehow caught my reservation without me saying anything, and he later asked his youngest sister, "Why is Father more supportive than Mother?" and I thought, Well, I guess Father doesn't really know what's involved! I was concerned about snowstorms and I realized babies aren't always born exactly when we plan them to be born, so I thought that they could have a long stay here. As it was, they came to spend Christmas with us on December 26th, and they said their baby would be born December 30th or 31st. They seemed very calm about everything, and the midwife came to our home to check us out and the surroundings where the baby would be born, and she didn't seem to think that the baby would be born quite that quickly, and as it turned out, rather than being born before the New Year, he was born January 24th. So they spent a whole month here.

During that time, our daughter-in-law gave up completely that a baby was going to be born, and I kept reassuring her that every baby that I knew of had come out, none had ever stayed in, but the night of the birth I realized that subconsciously I had also given up that this baby would ever be born, because I worked at Personal Care till eleven that night and came home and did some reading and probably fell asleep around midnight. At 2:30 in the morning our son was standing beside the bed holding Kholiswa and he said, we're in full labour upstairs, and would Dad try and keep Kholi asleep? My first thought when I saw my son in my bedroom was, what is he doing in my bedroom? My first thought was not, there's going to be a baby. So I must have given up by that time, too.

Anyway it turned out that it was a great experience. At first we just tolerated the idea of having a baby in our house, and when the midwife arrived, she had brought her one-year-old child along, and so I felt that my biggest duty was to keep her child out of her way so that she could do what she had to do. I sat in the living room trying to get her child back to sleep, and meanwhile our son came down and said to his father, "If you would like to be part of this, feel free to come upstairs." As it turned out, Wern was up there when the child was born and I was down here trying to get the midwife's baby back to sleep, but within minutes my husband came down and said, "It's a boy!" And I just dropped the midwife's baby on the floor [laughs] and ran upstairs, and we all sat on her bed. Vicki, who was expecting a baby a month later, had come too, and we all sat there and we were just rejoicing in the birth of this child, and then I realized I hadn't heard the baby cry. He was snuggled up right next to his mother, and finally I said, "Is that baby alive?" The midwife pulled it out and I realized, yes, it was alive, so then it was OK to have it snuggled up beside its mother, but I did want to make sure it was alive. And I had always thought there would be a lot of commotion with cutting the cord and all kinds of thing, and we just sat there for some time, just gloating over this birth, nobody was concerned about anything, and after a while the midwife said to my husband he could go and get the scissors up, which he had put in a pot to boil. [laughs] So he said, "You told me to boil them for half an hour, and it isn't half an hour yet," and she said, "Just go get them." So he went down to get the scissors and he handed them to our son, and he cut the cord. All this time we were sitting there in candlelight, and then our son said something about, what about the placenta? and the midwife said, "We shouldn't leave it too long, if it doesn't come we should do something." And he said, "Well what do they do in the hospital?" and she said, "Oh sometimes the doctor pulls it out!" Anyway, about half an hour later she decided we should do something, so they had Maggie get out of bed and squat over an ice cream pail, and the placenta did come out. And then the midwife and David walked into another room where there was more room to study the placenta, apparently they can see in the placenta whether the baby was full term or premature and there are other things they check the placenta for. But otherwise there were no drops put in his eyes or anything like that.

Sounds very peaceful.

It was. Of course by that time, I'm not sure what time it was, but we were all getting somewhat tired, so I went downstairs and I noticed Kholi stirring in our bed, so I picked her up and carried her upstairs and at that point she was clinging to Grandma very much, although usually she wanted to be with her parents. She sat on my lap and she was dazed from having been asleep, and her mother said to her, "The baby is not in my tummy any more. The baby is here." And she showed her the baby, and of course it didn't register. Then I picked up the baby so I was holding Kholi on my lap and I put the baby on her lap and we had been doing a lot of playing with where's your nose, where are your ears, so I said to her, "Does the baby have a nose?" So she touched the baby's nose, and I said, "Does the baby have ears?" so she touched the baby's ears, and then she put her finger on the baby's hand and the baby clasped her finger and I think from that moment she knew she had a brother.

Then, since we have quite a steep flight of stairs, I thought we'd bring Maggie all her meals up the first day or two, she just wasn't going to walk those stairs. Well, somehow we all got a few hours of sleep that night yet, and then I was having breakfast at around 8:30 or so, and I looked up, and there was Maggie with her newborn child coming down, and I said, "What are you doing down here!" and she said, "It was lonely up there." So I said, "Well, you're not going up and down those stairs." So she did stay downstairs that day, but the second day she was up and down the stairs. And by the third day they were packing up and leaving for Saskatoon. [laughs]

What reactions did you get?
I guess all through that was one thing that kind of bothered us, we couldn't openly talk about it, because, well, because people thought we were crazy, and actually after the baby was born, one of the staff people at the hospital where I work had said, "I knew they were strange, but I didn't know they were *that* strange!" [laughs] She meant David and Maggie. I thought David and Maggie could take it, so I told David that and he said, "She needs to have her horizons broadened." [laughs]

In a small community I think it is very hard to do something different like that.
People just really didn't believe it! That we had had a home birth! And if we had, then — by choice?!

Yes, I hear the same story from other people, their reactions to home births. — There are of course advantages and disadvantages of each, I guess.
Well, it's not something that you go into lightly. They had read up very very well, they were not tempting fate.

And she'd had one birth already, she knew what her chances were.
Yes. And actually she has very easy births, I mean the midwife got here just in time to catch the baby, and she probably could have had it without her.

Vicki Neufeld

Vicki Neufeld was born in Boissevain, Manitoba, in 1961. She and her husband, Ritchie Campbell, have three children. They farm near Minto, Manitoba. Vicki is my sister Elsa's daughter.

Elsa had told me about Vicki's experience with episiotomy during her first birth. I remember thinking in September 1994, when Vicki came to my house for an interview, that I would rather have a social visit that included her children than a discussion focussed on the pain of episiotomy. Within that story is the whole phenomenon of how we women forgive and forget our painful birth giving as long as we have a healthy baby in the end. It is hard to admit that I had gone out of my way to avoid hearing both the happy and sad stories even within my own family. Vicki moved from feeling victimized in her first birth giving to insisting on no episiotomy for her third birth.

An article entitled "Does Episiotomy Prevent Perineal Trauma and Pelvic Floor Relaxation?" by Michael C. Klein et al. discusses a scientific study of episiotomy conducted by a group of researchers at several Montreal hospitals and McGill University. It reports that women retaining an intact perineum (i.e., having no episiotomy) had the least perineal pain, and that women giving birth with an intact perineum fared best. The researchers recommended that the liberal or routine use of episiotomy be abandoned.

I WAS WHEELED DOWN to the labour room, and on the way down there I remember the doctor saying to my husband, "Well, if we hurry, this baby will be born before midnight." And at the time I thought, oh that'd be great, it had only been ten o'clock when I started, and if I could have this baby before midnight, all those horror stories of twelve-hour labours weren't for me. But in hindsight I often think, because I got to know that doctor later, he was in a hurry, he wanted things done fast, and if I was going to have this baby before midnight, then he would be on his own and he would be out of there! Anyway, in the labour room, I remember them telling me not to push until I was told to. And I never did have that urge to push, and I'm not sure if it was because everything was in such a rush and I never had control of my feelings, but I never actually had the urge to push until my third child. So I pushed — it wasn't very many times, I think maybe twice, three times I pushed, and then he said he was giving me an episiotomy, and it was over so quick, and hardly hurt at that time, that I never thought much about it. So Jenna was born two pushes later. It was very fast and very quick; I just remember feeling a total sense of relief, especially when they put that warm sheet on me — oh, it was heaven! And then he was stitching me up, and I remember lying there thinking of all the horror stories I had heard of women saying, oh they lay there for *hours* getting stitched up, and he had stitched me up before I would even have time to tie my shoes, and I thought, that's great, very little there, I'm in really good shape! Then the doctor said again to my husband, "Let's go down to the bar for a beer, because there's still time." And I didn't appreciate that. I had just had a baby, and this man was talking about going down to the bar for a beer, and I didn't like that. I went back to the room, and after that it was just a haze. I held Jenna and I slept, I guess. Right away I wanted to start nursing her, but that was kind of futile. So the next morning I was wanting to start nursing her, and both of us were having a lot of trouble.

Were your stitches bothering you?

Oh, yeah. That's a whole story in itself. The day after the birth it wasn't so bad, it was painful everywhere, and they were giving me Tylenol and sitz baths, it was the second day that I started complaining about them. The doctor came in to check the stitches, and I remember a nurse leaning over his shoulder taking a look, and she congratulated him on what a fine job he had done on the stitches. So it was later that day I figured — I remember a nurse coming in and saying when she had had her first baby, she had had the guts to actually have a look, to see what it looked like, so I figured OK, I'm going to ask her for a mirror. She gave me a mirror and I had a look, and I was absolutely horrified at what I saw. My breasts were swollen and my tummy was saggy, and then what was this! This was — I couldn't even imagine ever using that bottom end again! [laughs] It was just lumpy and swollen and red, and absolutely disgusting. Terrible. And then it was probably that night, the next morning, that it actually started burning when I urinated. I knew that wasn't right, that something was wrong. So then the other doctor, who hadn't delivered the baby, came in and had a look. He just said, "They've got to come out, you've got to have new ones. And this is going to hurt." So he gave me a couple of needles to freeze; well, that was *very* painful, and then he ripped out the stitches, and he did it again, and I was sent home an hour later. So that my recovery time — well, you could probably say I'm still recovering. But I had a recovery time, oh, of at least a month. I remember the public health nurse coming out, as they do after you've had your first child, and I was in my housecoat. And I remember I had a chicken in the oven. And she says, "Oh, you must be doing OK, you can get a meal together like that." It was much later when I thought she must have really wondered about me, because it was a couple of weeks after the birth, and I was still in my housecoat, and we're talking the middle of the day, but I didn't take that housecoat off, I didn't wear any underwear, any clothes, unless I was going out specially, in the evening, or for a special occasion, but I stayed in my housecoat, because it just hurt too much. And I'd have a heat lamp, grabbing a heat lamp from the barn, one we used to keep the cows warm, or the calves, hooking it up and just lying in front of this heat lamp, trying to dry out these stitches.

Did the doctor say anything about what was wrong with his first stitching?
No. He never ever came back to me and apologized, or gave any kind of excuse or reason.

Did you have him for the next baby too?
No. No. This other doctor was there again. And those stitches still bother me if I'm mentally overstimulated, or if I'm physically — that's where my, where it pains. So it's — it's very odd.

No, it's not odd, because there has been extreme trauma there, and it's stored in the body; maybe you can release it somehow.
Well I always say I never had trauma until I had children. [laughs] And not just the giving birth to them, it's the raising part, too. I never knew I had a temper until I had children. I had a different doctor for my other pregnancies, and I had expressed my concern from my first pregnancy, about the episiotomy, and could we do things differently. I had an episiotomy, but it was so insignificant to the first one that I barely recognized that, I guess because I didn't have time, either.

Landon was only twenty-four hours old, and he stopped responding — this is going to make me cry even to think about it. Within twenty-four hours he had caught viral pneumonia. So it was about five o'clock in the morning and the doctor had been called in, because he wasn't responding to the nurses any more. And the doctor came in and said that he would be rushed into Brandon, to the specialist there. So like I said, I didn't have time to think about my problems at that time. So whether my stitches were just as severe or not, really, I don't recall that.

Then with Morgan I had to worry the whole pregnancy, because I was only about eight weeks pregnant, and my sister and I had decided to go to Africa to see David, so I had to have all these immunizations. Only Tex and I knew at that time that I was pregnant, and I didn't even think! The public health nurse was administering these immunizations, and then she said, after, "You're not pregnant by any chance, are you?" My heart just fell.

And there again the episiotomy wasn't as traumatic as the first one.

I had no episiotomy with the third one. That's why I keep thinking this must have been a different doctor; isn't that terrible, I can't even remember the doctor! I had said to him that I'd been reading a lot and hearing a lot that through massage and other things an episiotomy really wasn't necessary as long as the doctor wasn't in a hurry and everything was fine with me. Well, I may have been in labour longer, but the actual pushing part — I pushed Morgan out in one and a half pushes. It was so quick, and the recovery time is just ninety percent faster when you have no episiotomy. It's just amazing to me that they will still do that to women. And I would say that to my friends later too, you just wouldn't believe the recovery time, how different it is without the episiotomy. Yes, I fought back about the episiotomy by my third child, but if it hadn't been for the doctor also wanting to support me, I would have had another episiotomy. When you're in labour and fighting to get this child out, you're very vulnerable, and the doctor makes the decisions. And I recommend that to all women giving birth, you've got to say it to them, over and over again, every time you have a visit with them, what your intentions are, and what you expect of them.

Gertrude Epp

Gertrude (Penner) Epp was born in 1900 in Tiegerweide, Russia. She and her husband, Bernhard, have eight children. They immigrated to Canada in 1924; in fact, Gertrude was expecting their first child at the time of their voyage. She has lived in St. Catharines, Ontario, and in Winnipeg and Boissevain, Manitoba. As they were recent immigrants and poor when they had their children, she and her sisters-in-law resourcefully learned to be midwives for each other. She left her parents behind in Russia, and it was years before she heard about their final days. The simple recounting of her experiences impressed on me how powerful the human voice is in storytelling.

[Translated from German]

When did you come to Canada from Russia?
We were married in '22, and in '24 we were leaving. And I was pregnant with my first child. I had a very bad crossing on the ship. [laughs] And so we arrived in Quebec. And from Quebec we drove to Toronto, and there we had to disembark, and there they already had the names of immigrants who would be arriving. And a Mr. Schneider came along, and he wanted to take us with him. He spoke no German, we spoke no English. It was in Waterloo, Ontario. He lived on a farm in Hamburg. So I asked him if there was any way I could earn some money. "Sure," he said, "you can come to

our house, my wife has just had a baby, and she needs some help." Yes — but only for one day a week. Do the laundry, that kind of thing, tidy the house. Yes, and I was that way myself. The milkman came by this farm every morning, by horse, to go to the city. So I drove with him in the morning and worked there, my husband was working on the road, the road was being built then, and in the evening the man would bring me home in his car. Finally I quit, it was August. And in January our daughter was born. And then I stopped with that.

Was she born at home or in the hospital?

No, we had a — here she's called a "midwife," yes? she had come from Russia too. And we had agreed that she was going to come. And our neighbour woman, who had no children, knew much more than I did. She asked me detailed questions. "Oh," she said, "at this and this time is when your baby will be born." OK. And so my husband got a horse and a sled, there was quite a bit of snow, and so he went to fetch the midwife. She came over, that was Saturday, and she wanted to have her family at her house on Sunday. And she said, "It won't happen yet." So he had to take her back home, and then three o'clock at night I said to my husband, "This is something different." Oh my, and so he had to get the horse hitched up to the sled again. And our neighbour woman came and stayed with me. And the pain was so strong already, it took so long before he — it was night, he had to go by sled — and the baby was born before the midwife got there! Everything went well. And it was cold, I wanted to tell her, "At least cover the baby up, it's too cold!" Finally I was able to show her with gestures, and she covered it up. And she stayed with me. And then when the midwife came she took care of everything and stayed with us for a whole week. She cooked for us — at that time we had to stay in bed. I never stayed in bed as long as others did. "I won't stay in bed any longer than one week!" I said. [laughs] How much my husband paid her I don't remember.

We had to promise, as immigrants, that we would go to the farm. My husband had a good job in the city by then, but because this promise had been made, we had to go to the farm in Whitewater [in Manitoba]. It was a big farm, oh I think we were thirteen families in all. That was '24. My baby was three weeks old. We didn't go with all the others, I couldn't go yet at that time. We went by train. My husband built a travel cradle to put the baby in. We arrived in Whitewater, there was no station, just an old train car. And there was no snow, but it was cold, frozen solid. And they came to get us from the farm in a hayrack. Oh my, I thought to myself, where have we come to now! So then we got there, and on the yard there was a big house where they took us in, and that's where we lived, four families, until all the land was divided up, and the houses were assigned. We didn't have one so we built a house, a small house and barn, and we moved there.

Can you tell me about your other births?
Yes. Annie was just one year and five months old, and then Ben came along. We were poor, none of us had any money, and we didn't have a telephone either. So my husband drove to the farm and phoned to Boissevain, to the doctor. And by the time the doctor came, Ben had already arrived. And so he looked after it. And that cost us thirty dollars! It was very difficult to get that much money together, for us on the farm at that time. In the beginning we just had a few cows, and one of us would milk them, and the milk was divided up between the families, a cup of milk for each person. But we had some money, we wanted to pay our travel loan. We bought a cow, and so at least we had some milk, we bought a few chickens, and where we lived there was a garage, and the garage was set up for us to live in, that's where Ben was born. And then later on the land was divided up and we got the section with no house on it. So then our house was built, and a barn, and that's where Heinz was born.

We had no money to pay a doctor again, so my sisters-in-law came over. The midwife had explained a lot to me when she was with me for a week. And so when Heinz was born, I had prepared everything: I boiled some twine and put it in a little box, poor as we were, and then I told the women how they were supposed to bind it and cut it off, and everything went just fine. I was the youngest of all of them, the family I had married into. So with Heinz we did it that way already, also with Gerhard, and with Gerdie, always without the doctor. Heinz, Gerhard, Gerdie, Jakob — oh yes, when I was pregnant with Jakob, that was the winter we also had scarlet fever. Oh, I had a difficult winter then. Oh my, that was hard! And then the last two. The doctor from Deloraine knew we couldn't afford the hospital, so he came over. And so he attended Mariechen's birth. And Selma I was in the hospital. Yes, by then we had a bit more money. [laughs]

What happened to your own family members, the ones who did not come to Canada?
Oh yes. They wanted to come too. We came with the first group, and they had papers to come with the fourth group. My father was sick, he had a heart disease. And so they weren't able to leave with their group in August, and that was the end of it. He died in September. My sisters were all still unmarried then, they married later, when I was already here. And then when the Germans were in Russia, they tried to get our Mennonite people into Germany. That was already after World War II. And then they got to

Poland, and from there the Germans wanted to bring them to Germany. And then the Russians came, and took them back and sent them to Siberia. They built up these wagons with a roof over top, and that is how my poor mother travelled, with horses. Some people died, and they had to be buried along the way, and just keep going, keep going, and the horses got tired, when it was muddy, they would almost get stuck, and that's how my poor mother — but she did make it to Poland, and then they were sent to Siberia, and there she starved to death. They had so little to eat, and my sister said she died of weakness. Yes. And they had nothing. They got one bread, bread cost a hundred dollars. And so they cut the bread in ten pieces, and sold one slice for ten dollars, to get some money. And then for that money they hired someone to dig a grave for my mother. And those three sisters went and buried — [voice breaks] Yes. They had it hard, very hard.

Did you receive the news right away?
No. For a time we got no news at all, because of the Second World War. Then all of a sudden we got news. Now we write each other. I visited my niece in Germany last year. She told me a lot about their experiences there.

Agatha Martens

Agatha (Schroeder) Martens was born in 1917 in Arkadak, Russia. When she was six and a half years old she came with her parents, Johann and Anna, to Canada and lived in the Manitoba communities of Winnipeg, Steinbach, Niverville, and Morris, and since 1932 again in Winnipeg. She and her husband, Abram, had five children. Agatha Martens worked as a housemaid when she first came to Canada, and when her husband was ill she went to work again as a waitress and as a store clerk at Simpsons Sears.

As a child, Agatha experienced the Russian Revolution and the immigration to Canada. Like many other young immigrant women, both Mennonite and non-Mennonite, Agatha worked as a domestic. At the age of fourteen, when other girls her age went to school, she worked to pay the family's Reiseschuld *(travel debt). The immigrants of the 1920s had been so impoverished by the war and the revolution that most could not pay their transportation costs. The Mennonites in Canada formed an organization that collectively took on the debt owed to the Canadian Pacific Railway until the immigrants could earn the money to repay it.*

The Mädchenheim *(girls' home) Agatha refers to in her story was a supportive "home away from home" in Winnipeg, where the young women who worked as maids could go on their day off. The housemother kept an eye on them.*

Later in life Agatha kept a journal in which she worked out problems in living and in understanding behaviour, her own and others'. Her conflict about whether to destroy the journals so as not to hurt anyone's feelings or to leave them as one woman's honest record of her life is understandable.

What are your earliest memories of Russia?
Of course my first memories are kind of bad memories. You know, those were bad years. In the first place we had to leave Arkadak, my dad was teaching there, but things were getting harder and harder, so they decided to move back to Rosental, where Grandpa Schroeder lived. I remember standing in line, waiting for a shirt. I was very shy, and this lady spoke a very correct German. We also spoke High German, but I was afraid of her. And then if you got this shirt, you were supposed to go to Kindergarten, which for some reason or other I didn't want to do. And so I would hide, I remember this being a big problem, because we desperately needed things.

I also remember some of the things about Dad being taken away, how upset everyone was. Dad would not be back, he was supposed to be shot. That was very traumatic. I must have been about four when Dad came back, and my auntie reminded me later how I had said, "Do you remember how we all prayed, and you said if my dad got out again, we would all remember to thank God?" Of course in the joy of seeing Dad again, everybody forgot about God. And I reminded them.

Getting ready to go to Canada. The preparations were made, baskets of roasted buns, the good-byes, too, because Grandma Schroeder and the aunties, widows whom we lived with at the time, were not coming yet. It was people standing at the station crying, and not knowing, are we really going to get out of here, and what's it going to be like. A child senses that, too. I remember it must have been the last Christmas in Russia, we didn't even have enough food, and my dad tried to make some little gifts from nothings, which I think pleased us children no end.

Do you remember anything of the trip itself?
We transferred in Liverpool to a bigger ship. My mother all this time was desperately seasick, she couldn't lift her head up. And my older sisters, who were teenagers, I'm sure wanted to enjoy themselves, but they had to look after us little ones. There was my brother John, just a year younger than I, and Erika was the baby, she was I think two years old, and she was crying for Mother. And I remember the different foods, we were hungry, yes, but the foods were different, the coffee had sugar in it. I remember the people saying, oh, coffee with sugar! And marmalade. We weren't used to marmalade. We maybe had jam, I suppose, but not marmalade.

I had very bad earaches on the ship, and in Liverpool I was taken to a Red Cross hospital. I can see the Red Cross nurses today as very stiff, uniforms or whatever, and I was taken there to get my ears treated, but I was very afraid. I thought, this is it, they're going to leave me here, they're going to go on. I don't know whether I cried, but I just remember this terrible fear; I had heard of children being left, and here they're going to leave me and go on to Canada without me.

Then we got onto a bigger ship, and I remember getting to Halifax. It had been hard, as I say, with Mother, she wasn't very strong as it was, because in Russia, when there was no bread, if we would come crying and saying, "We're hungry," Mother would usually have something in her big apron pocket, and she would go and get it out and give it to us children. Later on I thought of it, that was her bread! That was her ration. And she gave it to us, like mothers would. But anyway, she was run down. Just before we left she had had twins who died, and this must have all been very, very hard on her. But we children didn't realize that, we were demanding. We were hungry, and we'd come crying, and she'd give her food to us! So the ship should have been heavenly for us, but it was different food. This food was not cooked by our mother, it was different, it was not Mennonite food.

And then getting to Halifax, and riding the train, seems to me it was three days that we were on the train. I remember getting here to Winnipeg, sitting in that immigration hall on those hard benches. It was July, it was hot, we were probably very dirty, and waiting for relatives, who probably didn't know exactly when we would arrive.

And how heavenly it was, finally, to be put into a little home, somewhere on the farm. It seemed very desolate at the time, no trees, nothing around. People were very good to us though, people brought things. I always remember how grateful and thankful my parents were, saying how beautiful it was in Canada, that we could go to bed and not even lock the doors — in those days that was possible — and go to sleep and not worry about somebody pounding on your door, taking out the men, or things like that.

I didn't start school until I was nearly eight. We were taught at home, though, which I've always been thankful for. My father taught us to read and write German, he insisted on it, and taught other children who used to come round. He had been a teacher, and he wanted us to learn German, not to forget it, which I am thankful for. I still can read anything, and write. So I owe that to my father. That was on the farm, those were hard years, too, things were not easy. He wasn't a farmer, and things just didn't seem to work out.

Then they decided to move to Winnipeg. We lived on William Avenue, in a big house. I still see the house and I often feel like saying, can I come in and look, we lived here once. But I haven't. We children *didn't* like the city. Oh we didn't like it. We weren't understood, we were made fun of. My mother wouldn't let me cut my hair. I was twenty-three when I cut my hair, and then I hadn't asked permission, and got reprimanded for that. But I had long braids and Canadian girls didn't wear braids those days, and my mother said I had to have braids, and so braids it was! And our clothes were made fun of. We were very unhappy here in Winnipeg. My biggest happiness was, across William Avenue where we lived was a library, and I used to go, and I found out that I could go into this library whenever I wanted to, I could go in and read books. And so of course whenever I could sneak away from work or from chores that Mother had for me, or looking after little Frieda — a little sister born here in Canada — then I would go and read books, and I loved that. People just didn't understand us, we were different, our language, I think.

I stopped school at fourteen, and went to work at what was then called nursemaid here in Winnipeg. Maybe you would call it babysitting now, although it was much more than that. I had to look after the children, I got five dollars a month for that, and uniforms, which saved me buying clothes, and of course my board and room, which meant a great deal. Four dollars at least every month went to Mom and Dad, because that would buy just about a hundred-pound sack of flour. Dad tried to earn a little bit of money here and there, but it was very hard, trying to eke out a living in those days. I worked my way up, and later on got twenty, even thirty dollars a month, but I started with five dollars a month. I often cringe inside when I see my grandchildren these days who are just handed money like that, or their allowance is five dollars a week or something — my goodness.

You mentioned that your parents had fifteen children, but only seven remained alive.

This all happened in Russia. And most of them died in infancy. My mother had twins twice. I remember about the first twins — they were born before I was — that the little girl, Magdalena, was much stronger, and her brother, Peter, got dysentery, those days there was no control over it. It was summertime, and then she got it and they both died within days. They had been healthy, happy babies, but it happened very quickly. I remember my mother saying, "I could always get over it, I could somehow find solace, but your dad was heartbroken when children died and we had to bury them." They were then nine months old. You know, babies at nine months are so cute, I often wonder, how did they cope with all that! I haven't buried a child in my life, I hope I never will, and they buried so many. The twins that were born just before we came to Canada, they were very tiny, they were born in an unheated hospital, and Mother was so run down, and had been so hungry, she couldn't nurse them, she had no milk. There was no milk available, so they made some kind of sweet tea and dropped it into their mouths to try and keep them alive. I think they died of malnutrition, and Mother said, "We have to thank God for that, we didn't know how we were going to manage." And so they were gone. That's four children, so in between were some more. I remember my sister Anna dying at the age of twelve of meningitis, and that was very, very tragic for all of us. I don't remember her very well, she'd been older and worried about us, the younger ones, she had helped look after us. She asked our parents to make sure that we would be all right and to watch us, before she died. I remember her funeral. Things were hard then already, I guess, and Mother decided that Anna should have a dress out of her own wedding dress. Mother was a good seamstress, she made the dress, and that's the way she was buried.

I remember years after, when Mom and Grandma would talk about Nyuta, as they call her, that's Anna, that I was jealous, because I thought, Nyuta must have been an angel, she must have been so perfect, the way they talked about her, and here was I, I thought of myself as an ugly duckling, and I always thought, why did a beautiful girl like that have to die? How could God do that, how could he take a beautiful girl like that when I'm still living? [laughs]

So many people died. I remember us all being very sick with typhoid fever, we all had it, we all lost our hair, we were full of sores. I remember crying and crying because my mouth and everything was so sore, I guess it was from malnutrition too. Little Grandma Schroeder, she was a very tiny woman, who lived to be ninety-six years old, never got typhoid fever, she went around looking after everybody. We were all living together in Rosental, in that house with Grandpa, in that typhoid fever epidemic. The women seemed to be stronger than the men, because Grandpa Thiessen died, Grandpa Schroeder died, all my aunts were widowed at the time, their husbands died, yet little Grandma Schroeder, who was not very strong, she survived!

Changing the subject, how did you meet your husband?
I met him at a wedding, I remember it very well, I saw him and we sort of took to each other right away. He was a big man, he was over six feet tall, and I'm not five feet tall, we were friends right away, we dated — we did not see each other every day, I worked in Winnipeg then as a housemaid, and I only got off every Thursday afternoon, and every other Sunday. We always went to the girls' home, the *Mädchenheim*. The lady of the house would let you take a bag lunch, the housemother would make tea and coffee for us and sometimes even soup. We girls would meet in Eaton's and look around

and shop, then go to the girls' home. After we had had our lunch and our Bible study with one of the ministers, we sang. We sang so many beautiful songs. Then the boys would come and get us, and we might go out. What did we do? Go for a walk, or they would walk us home, all the way from Bannatyne Avenue to Academy Road somewhere out in River Heights, or Tuxedo, where we worked, that was our day off. They were good days. Yes, we had a lot of good friends in the home, and we would talk to each other, tell our problems — of course we had problems, we certainly did! We supported each other. We were all in the same boat, we were all poor — and the funny thing is that we never thought of ourselves as poor! I remember, though, also the loneliness. And I'm prone to that anyway. I was desperately lonesome sometimes for the family. And Morris, where my parents lived at the time, was just forty miles away. *But.* Those days we just didn't go home just like that, on your day off. That was unheard of!

And you started working from the age of fourteen, so you were quite young.
Right. Yes, I was young, but I must say, I was very fortunate. My sister, who was ten years older than I was, also worked here, and she took me under her wing. And I was very naïve, very — I didn't know some things — I don't know whether I should mention this here about how when you work in houses like that, things happen. This one man was forever — I didn't know what was going on, because every time he'd go by he'd — until I said to my sister, "I don't like this, I don't know what's going on," and she said, "What?" and then she got Miss Epp, and Miss Epp knew right away, she said, "You're not staying there!" She would make sure that you got a good place, and so most of the time you did. I thank God for her.

You had to work hard, some places you got up at 6:30 in the morning, and you were downstairs by seven o'clock, you would get the gentleman's breakfast, he'd be off to work; the lady of the house would be in bed very often till noon, you had to bring her breakfast in bed! And then you looked after the children, you got them off to school, or whatever the case was. Yes, and you worked from seven till seven for sure, if not longer. In some of the homes you were really treated well, you had your own room, which was heavenly to us, because there you could go and close the door. I remember one time being very sick, I had pneumonia, and they got their own doctor — there was no such a thing as medicare, *I* couldn't pay for it — to come in and he prescribed medicine, they paid for it, they looked after me, they were wonderful to me.

You said earlier, "Childbirth is an experience that totally changes you."
That's right. Well, it changed me. I felt this terrible sense of — here's a little human being, you brought him into the world, you're responsible. What

are you going to do with it? I felt very deeply about the responsibility, and my children I don't think know this, I don't know whether I've ever told them in detail — we have dedication in our church, I think most churches have it now — but I used to dedicate my children when I'd first get them in the hospital, look at this little miracle that happened again, and used to just turn them over to the Lord and say, "I'll do my best, but I'll make mistakes. I know I will, and I'll maybe do things wrong. You have to help me." I didn't like being pregnant, I was terribly big, I was very clumsy, but once my children were there, I had it made. It didn't matter, I just loved them so terribly much. I always thought I was going to have a dozen children, but after the twins, I was thirty-six, and I had a hard time, the doctor had said that I couldn't have another baby. He called in the specialist, and they didn't know about twins then yet, and he said, no you can't carry this, you won't carry it!

Oh, they didn't know you had twins?

No, at the beginning they didn't know. And I said, "Well, that's all right. If I won't carry, I'll go home, and if I lose the baby" — they wanted me to — well, I don't know, I was in the hospital, this was at the beginning of the pregnancy, and I had problems, and they just didn't think that I could carry that baby. And I said, "Well, I'm going home, and I'll do my best, and if I lose it, I'll accept it as such, but I won't let you do anything, I must carry on." And so I did. I kept on saying to the doctor, "My mother said she always felt terrible when she was carrying twins; am *I* carrying twins?" and he said, "Oh, don't talk about twins!" And then he noticed the two heartbeats, those days they didn't do ultrasounds yet, and he said, "At the end of your pregnancy we'll x-ray." They x-rayed — my girls are horrified at that now, but they did. He said, "I'll phone you when the results come." So he said to me, "Are you sitting down?" I said, "I don't need to be," and he said, "It is twins," and I said, "Yes, that's what I thought," and I had two big girls over seven pounds. And later on I went to that specialist and took my girls and showed them to him, I said, "I want you to see my twins." And he said, "If anybody had said that you could have one healthy baby, I would have said no." I said, "Well, I had great faith, I believed that if God wanted me to have that baby, He would help me through it."

How were the births?

The births were very hard, very difficult. I know several times they talked about Caesarean section, which they didn't do, I was always so anemic after. But I was always in the hospital at least for ten days, I always got a good rest. And one thing I was very fortunate, I'd always spring back. I was just so happy having the babies. I always thought, I can cope with anything as along as they're all right. And it was hard, especially after the twins, I had three older ones, Ed was then twelve, Marlene was ten, Richard was seven, but they all had to help — it was 1953 when our twins were born, it was a polio year, the children went to school late. For me that was a blessing, I think, because Marlene, my daughter of ten then, helped a great deal with those babies. And so did the boys, they all had to jump in and help with the chores.

Did you breast-feed your babies?
No. No, that's one thing I regret very much. I had problems right with the first baby, my breasts — I landed back in hospital three times because of my breasts. And so the doctor took me off, said don't try, and I tried again, but I wasn't successful at that. I see the young generation, my daughters all breast-feed, I admire them for it.

When your husband got sick, you went to work. Was this when your children were small?
The twins were seven years old at the time. I thought they were very young yet. My husband had to stay home six months, which was devastating for us, because we didn't have any money saved. We just made do from day to day, made our payments, and didn't make any debts, like good Mennonites, but just lived from day to day. But we had very good friends who helped us out at the time. I went back to work, and of course I said to my husband, "I'll only go as long as you can't work." I think I made seventy-five cents an hour at that time. But imagine seventy-five cents, how much was that going to help? with buying groceries for seven people. But it did, I guess. I worked in a little restaurant, and I'd run back and forth, those hours that the children were at school, and at noon my husband was there, when Catherine and Caroline would come home. But I never stopped working. I kept right on. In the first place, I must say, I liked it! I was also in those days a very pernickety housekeeper, and my husband did help, but you know, like Mennonite men. . . . I got on at Sears later, and I liked working there, and due to ill health — I was only working part-time — I often had to quit in between and stay home for a little while, but I always went back.

Did you have a sense of independence?
Oh, very much so! Just to be able to know — and I'm not running my husband down, I don't want to do that, he just did what he was used to, I guess, but I had very little money. I never got money in my hands. Because my husband did the grocery shopping, which was very good, I appreciated

that a great deal, because I didn't drive. And here all of a sudden I had money in my hands. I loved it. I'm very happy these days, the way we seniors have money to spend and to give, and so I liked it very much, I never stopped working then, kept on as long as I could. I don't consider just because I don't work for pay any more that I've stopped working. I do a lot of volunteer work now. I love working for the MCC [Mennonite Central Committee]; we have a meal program downstairs, I help with that; and I belong to a ladies' aid.

You talked last time about keeping a journal and how that helps you to stay balanced or work out your problems.
Well, I think as I told you last time, I used to do that, I think they date back from 1960, something like that, when due to ill health I was housebound a lot of the time, and I was plagued with depression. I was very depressed sometimes. And so instead of running to people, or running to my minister, or whatever, I would write, jot it down. And it seemed to help me, it was my way of coping. I'd read them over again and wonder if I should chuck them. But I don't write very much any more. Somehow or other I found a very intimate Bible study, I found friends that I could really talk to, and I guess I don't need it as much. There are some things that, if they bother me very much, I'll go and jot it down.

I get a warm feeling listening to you. All our experiences are similar in some ways, especially raising children. As you said, childbirth changes you.
Oh, it changes you! I don't think anything in my life has changed me as much as the birth of a child. Oh, it's hard to watch them make mistakes, and then — now I see though, I think lo and behold, you know, sometimes I wish my husband could have lived a little longer to see how successful my children have been, what they've done with their lives. And I'm proud of them, very proud of them.

Agatha Warkentin

Agatha (Neufeld) Warkentin was born in 1943 in Deloraine, Manitoba. She and her husband, Bob, have two children. Agatha is a music teacher. I also interviewed her daughter, Robyn Epp. Our interview took place on Bob and Agatha's farm near Meadows, Manitoba, a comfortable drive into the country from Winnipeg. Agatha has been my friend since my husband and I moved to Winnipeg in 1966 and both our families had small children. I drove out to Agatha's home alone on a beautiful summer day, and we had tea in her kitchen with a view to the east and south of Meadows. We were surprised at how many feelings about motherhood we had never discussed, perhaps understandably since we met mostly in social situations with our husbands.

Women of our age are expected to know about pregnancy and labour and birth, because we grew up in the "modern" era. When you first found out you were pregnant, Agatha, how did you feel?

First of all, it seemed to be a very natural thing to be married and suddenly get pregnant. Now when I look back, I didn't even really think about birth control — it just seemed natural that I suddenly was pregnant. I remember thinking, well there goes my music out the window, because music means an awful lot to me. I remember telling my mother-in-law that I was pregnant. I went and played piano in her house, and she came in and said to me, "Are you sorry that you're pregnant?" and I wasn't really sorry, it was just that there was that conflict between my music and being pregnant. And when I got married there was no thought of going to university after you're married, that was taboo. I had always wished I could go to university to finish my music.

How did you resolve this?
Actually I found out I didn't have to give up music. I kept on teaching, and worked my family into my teaching career. My husband supported me a lot, and probably my children maybe have resented it that I was teaching, but I always taught in my home. And that was part of my life.

No different really than a farmer's wife who goes out to milk the cows at a certain time, the children have to live without her for a few hours.
Yes, yes, that's right. It's no different. And when I got pregnant with Richard, well, we just wanted another child. We thought it was not quite fair to have just one child, we wanted another child. And then that was it, no more children after that! [laughs]

So you were the oldest in the family, and you had been used to children in the family?
The year before I got married, I lived at home, and my mother started having foster children. That's when she got this little baby, and I remember having to take care of this little baby, which now I look back, really did help me a lot, I didn't feel insecure about taking care of Robyn. I knew how to make a formula, I knew how to wash diapers, to some extent, and just felt quite comfortable with that. But my mother is the one who helped me with that.

Both of your children were born in the hospital. Was it a good experience?
Yes, actually Robyn's was a very easy birth. I had an easy pregnancy. I was sick the first few months, which maybe is just a normal thing, morning sickness for three months, and then after that I had a very easy pregnancy. Well I should say I did have my appendix out when I was about five months pregnant. I'd had trouble with my appendix all my teenage years, but never to the extent that they had to remove it, and I remember going to the doctor, I guess for a physical, and the next day being violently ill, thinking I was having a miscarriage, because I was so innocent about the whole pregnancy, I really wasn't told very much. You know, when you're nineteen — in fact I don't even remember reading any books! When I think of what my daughter read compared to what I read! And Bob thinking, no, you're not having a miscarriage, it sounds like appendix. So we went in, we were

in the hospital at ten o'clock, and by 10:30 I was on the operating table. And the operation was very successful, I bounced back very quickly, and two weeks later I was just feeling my old self.

I remember wanting to wear maternity clothes so badly. But I just didn't show, it was frustrating! [laughs] When I went to prenatal classes, all these other women were wearing maternity clothes and looked so obviously pregnant, and I still walked in in ordinary clothes, and they kept saying, "You're not pregnant!" So finally I just put on maternity clothes so that I could say that I was pregnant. And when I did have Robyn, I remember this lady phoned me and she said, "Well, that was certainly a surprise!" And I said, "What do you mean?" "Well, you had your baby so early!" And I said, "No, my baby was a full-term baby," it was just that I had small children, Robyn was only four pounds twelve ounces. So it was a very easy birth.

Was the labour long?
It started in the morning — actually I woke up not feeling well, just feeling ill. And I had been at the doctor, and he had said, "Well, you could have your child any time." We went to Winnipeg — well, because we lived a good hour from the doctor, we felt we should be in the hospital sooner, and because it was my first birth, we didn't know exactly how things would go. Robyn was born at 4:30 in the afternoon, so it wasn't a long labour. Some people talk about having a really difficult, painful labour, and as far as I can remember it wasn't — I guess painful, but nothing out of the ordinary.

Did you have to have anesthesia of any sort?
No, none at all. I didn't have to have an episiotomy, nothing. Very natural birth. And because I had taken the prenatal class, I knew how to do the breathing, and it was just a very natural birth. Dr. Peter Friesen was my doctor. I trusted him and he was excellent with me. He was there the whole time.

Well, you were of course having your baby at the right time, in the daytime!
Yes, that's right! [laughs] 4:30 in the afternoon. But, no, he was there the whole time. I can't remember the nurses too much with Robyn. I guess they were there, in and out. I remember Bob had to do some business downtown, and he didn't realize though meanwhile that I had landed up in the delivery room, and he walked in and they all just — I remember hearing his voice, and the nurses saying, "What are you doing here!" and I said, "That's my husband, it's OK, he can come in." But at that time the men weren't allowed in, which is unfortunate in a way; sometimes I wish Bob had been there, and yet it hasn't hindered any relationship between us and

our children. I sometimes think, how do the women do it, they're so busy listening to the doctor giving the instructions how to deliver, and if you happen to have a husband who's very sensitive, you'd be concerned with him, too. It could be a hindrance. Yet on the other hand, the husband could really help a lot too. But I have no feelings about that, no regrets or any other, because at that time it just was that way. If I had a baby now — I don't know if I'd ask my husband to be there or not, I really don't.

With Richard I had a very unfortunate thing happen to me just six weeks before he was born. We were renovating our kitchen, and my husband had put the stove on wood blocks, so that he could put the plywood underneath the stove, and we didn't have running water at the time, so I had heated a kettle of water to wash my dishes. I'd made fried potatoes for dinner, and when I took the cast iron frying pan and put it towards the back of the stove, it tipped somehow, and all this scalding water poured over my body. And I remember just — well, I guess, yeah, screaming, and Bob quickly took my clothes off, and because at that time I was wearing a maternity girdle, the water stayed on my body quite a bit, so I was burnt quite badly on my right side. I said, "Oh, I'll be OK," but Bob realized that it was definitely more than just a light scalding. We phoned Bob's parents, and they came to get us. It was beastly cold, and all I could think of was to put on a clean sheet, a cotton sheet, so they wrapped me up in that and we went to the hospital. I stayed in the hospital overnight, because I was quite badly scalded. And I remember them monitoring me very, very closely, because I was at that point eight months pregnant.

So we stayed with my in-laws then for two weeks, and meanwhile I had to go to the doctor every other day for changing my bandages, and we were home two weeks, and then Richard was born on the 16th of February. I think it was about ten days early — and I think they were more concerned with that birth, I still hadn't healed completely, I had one scar that was very bad, and that was painful. With his birth I knew what to expect already, so it was a little different, and again it wasn't a difficult birth. I remember being in the labour room, and my doctor was curling, he's an avid curler, and this was close to midnight. And they were saying they were waiting for the doctor, and I said, "You know, I think you should call the doctor, because it's time for this baby to be born." And I must have had a nurse that either worked strictly by the book or had just graduated, because she said, "Oh no, Mrs. Warkentin, your baby isn't going to be born for a long time." And I said, "I know this baby is going to be born very shortly! You better get the doctor, get me into that delivery room!" And then an older nurse came in and she said, "Get this woman into the delivery room!" By then the doctor came, and I remember he was very upset that they hadn't called him sooner, because I was ready to deliver that baby.

I was very tired. That afternoon I had had this strange urge to finish things. I remember saying I was so tired, I couldn't push any more. And then they did give me some gas, but not very much. And I also remember them saying, "You have to push harder, or we're going to have to use forceps." I have a great fear of forceps, and I said, "No, don't use forceps, I'll keep on pushing." And I did. But I was born with forceps, and I'm wondering if that's maybe why I felt that way, I just did not want to have them — and yet, I guess if you have to have them, it can help. So both my children actually were not difficult births. I remember thinking when they said, "You have a boy!" I said, "Good, now we have one of each, and I don't have to go through this again." [laughs] I had no desire to have any more children after that. Oh, there was later on in life, but basically I felt, we had a girl and a boy, and we just didn't really think about having any more children.

Where was Robyn while you were in labour, where was she staying?
Robyn was with her Grandma Warkentin. We had prepared Robyn quite well that Mommy would have to go to the hospital, and she would have to stay with Grandma for a while, and when we came home we would have a baby. And then of course I landed up in the hospital with my scalding, and we came home, and the first thing she asked was, "Where's the baby?" Well, how are you going to explain to a two-year-old that there *is* no baby? She wasn't even quite two — she was twenty-two months — there *is* no baby. And she refused to have anything to do with me, she ignored me — mind you there was no way I could physically take care of her, I just couldn't. She was very upset that this baby wasn't there. But when Bob came to get me, she was with us, and when we came home, she did act a little peculiar, and finally we just took this baby upstairs and we spent the afternoon playing with her and letting her know that she was still loved very much, and we never had any jealousy with her or anything, she accepted the baby and I can't remember her being rough with the baby, or poking the baby or anything. I let her help me bathe the baby, and let her feel very important for a two-year-old. And it worked out OK, I think. [laughs]

I don't remember my mother being pregnant — oh, it just wasn't talked about! I was twelve years old, and I didn't realize my mother was pregnant. I remember the girls in school teasing me that my mother was pregnant again, and I think I beat them up, I was so upset, [laughs] because my mother hadn't told me, and how did *they* know something that I hadn't been told? And then going home and confronting my mother with this and her saying, "Well, yes, we are going to have a baby." Would have been easier maybe if my mother had been more open, but — I think it was difficult for them. It was kept so hush hush.

How was nursing, was it easy to get established?

With Robyn, I had no difficulty nursing. I nursed her for six weeks. The doctor encouraged me to nurse her, but because she was such a small baby, he felt she needed more protein, which now I really doubt, but anyway, at six weeks she had to have a little bit of meat every day. Now when I look back, why did she have to have this meat — it was a tiny, tiny amount, the tins dried out way before they were empty, but he just felt she needed protein. And gradually I put her on the bottle, and at six weeks I stopped nursing.

Richard I nursed, again I didn't have much difficulty nursing, but he was so hungry all the time. I nursed him for two weeks, and my milk just didn't seem to satisfy him. And then I got sick, and my breasts got very engorged, and I was kind of worried that maybe I was having breast fever. Actually it turned out I had the flu, but I didn't know that. So we rushed to the doctor, because I was not feeling well, and Richard wasn't eating, and I said to the doctor, "Give me milk formula for him, so that if I decide to stop nursing I have this formula." We went home to Bob's mom and dad's, and decided to stay there for night, and two o'clock this baby is crying, and finally I said to Bob, "This is it." I went and made him a formula, and he took the formula better than he took my breast milk, so I just stopped nursing. And after that I didn't have this hungry baby any more. So I don't know, was it that my milk just wasn't strong enough, or was I not relaxed enough, I don't know. But I nursed him for two weeks. I can't say I particularly enjoyed nursing. I don't know why. I know when Robyn was nursing her children, she enjoyed it so much. I enjoyed holding them and giving them the bottle, but I'm not that patient.

I nursed Robyn till the end of June. Maybe another reason I stopped nursing, all my friends were getting married that summer. And I couldn't picture myself going to all these weddings with this baby and nursing. Twenty-four years ago you were a little more embarrassed about nursing than you are now.

Oh yeah, it was much more difficult, in public, anyway.

Much more difficult, yeah. We were invited to all these weddings, and I had wonderful people who were thrilled to babysit this little baby! And it was one way of not having to worry about the nursing part. — With Richard, Bob was very supportive, he took care of Robyn the whole time, and because he was born in February, he had two, three months to really help, I remember the whole family around the table while I was bathing Richard, and Bob watching with Robyn, and it was a real family unit.

Did you have any household help?
Bob's sister, Marlene, helped a lot. She would come on a Saturday and watch the children for me when I did my housework. She wasn't married at the time, and she would come up Saturday afternoon, with fresh *Zwieback* (rolls) or something, and then she would watch the kids for me and I would be able to do my housework. Bob's sister and mother came and made my garden for me the first year, simply because they felt I wasn't strong enough to do this after having a baby. And after Richard, again, Marlene was really supportive. She was going to Westgate [Mennonite Collegiate], and she would bring her friends home and they would come on Saturday and babysit for us, and I would be able to do my own work then. And that's about all the help I had.

Did you feel it was enough? Could you have used more?
I physically was capable of doing it, so I never considered having help. I managed without. It just seemed natural that I could do these things. If it didn't get done I [laughs] probably got upset with my husband and said, let's get this done!

Did you know that if you needed somebody, you had family to call upon for an emergency?
Yes, I could really depend on Bob's mom. She was wonderful. I remember once during seeding time I got the flu. There was no way I could take care of these two children, and Bob had to go on the land, and we just phoned Bob's mom, and she took care of the kids that day for me. My mother-in-law was a very big support. Very understanding. And often, if we wanted to go to Winnipeg, she would keep one of the children. That really helped. I also had a wonderful neighbour who babysat a lot for us, and who often came over and just talked, and was encouraging, and would bring something for the kids; she was just a wonderful neighbour. She was the same age as my mother, so I had a very difficult time at first, calling her Helen. Because we'd been taught that people that age were Mrs. or Aunt or whatever. But we formed a very, very good friendship, and she was really supportive in that way. So that's the type of help I had.

DI BRANDT

Di (Janzen) Brandt was born in 1952 in Winkler and lived in Reinland, Manitoba, before attending university in Winnipeg and Toronto. She has two daughters. Di is a well-known poet, writer, and teacher. She has published four books of poetry (two of which were nominated for the Governor General's Award) and two books of non-fiction.

I first talked to Di about my project at a graduate-school dance where we strained to hear each other over loud music. She was interested to know that I was finding older Mennonite women who would answer my questions. Di discussed seven of the interviews in her Ph.D. dissertation and in the published book version of it, Wild Mother Dancing: Maternal Narrative in Canadian Literature.

THE THING I REMEMBER as being most significant is that it was a very double experience, becoming pregnant and having children. I had my first child just after I finished my master's degree in English at University of Toronto, and it was like moving into a different kind of experience altogether. It had nothing to do with the studies that I'd been doing. I'd been reading all this literature which was supposed to have something to do with real life. Most of the stuff I'd been reading was Romantic poetry by English men, and so on, and it was suddenly totally irrelevant. I was really shocked by this, how completely different this experience was, and how unprepared I was for it.

I remember this wonderful thing that happened: my centre changed from being inside my head to being in my belly. It was just wonderful, the centre of gravity shifted, you know. I just loved being pregnant, loved getting really big and awkward and sort of sailing along the street, and I loved living so much in my body. That was a new thing for me, because I lived in my head so much before that. It was the first time I ever felt like that, I felt totally grounded and part of the earth, and it was great. I didn't have a lot of language for it, although I'm a very language-oriented person. The stories that I had in my head didn't have anything to do with this experience, so that was really weird, intellectually it felt like falling into this hole, this void. But the experience in my body was just wonderful.

The other thing was that while I felt so relaxed and physical, there was this whole bureaucracy at the hospital. That was really difficult for me, I'd never been in a hospital before, and I was totally terrified by it. I did all this reading about childbirth while I was pregnant, and I was really prepared, I think. But my doctor and the whole hospital experience was so different from what I was reading and what I wanted it to be. I felt quite numbed by the hospital experience and the way I was treated there.

Had you talked to your doctor about it at all?

Well, a little bit, but we didn't have a very chatty relationship. He was very businesslike, he just rushed me through. Mostly just gave me a hard time about gaining too much weight all the time. It was not a terribly pleasant relationship, and I was really naïve about that system. I didn't know how to find a better doctor, and I didn't know really what kind of choices there were. This was, after all, supposed to be the progressive place and everything. And then he was on holidays when it actually happened, so I had this other doctor, whom I had never met. I went into labour on a Sunday night, and there was nobody else in the labour section of that hospital, so there were at least a dozen or more attendants in the room. They were all in my room, because there were no other people there.

I don't understand, why were they all there?

Well, because it was like sort of this whole staff of the labour section. You know, if there had been five women in labour, they would have been spread out over five women, but because I was the only one there — it was really bizarre, I was just lying on this table and every time I looked around there was another person, I was surrounded! I told them when I went in that I didn't want to have any medication, and the nurse that was registering me laughed and said, "Everybody says that when they come in, you better sign because everybody wants it in the end." So that was the beginning of the intimidation. And I had a really short labour, it was three hours long, and it was not very difficult, but they made me have an epidural, which I really resent, still. I was already on the table, the head was starting to come out, there was absolutely no need for an epidural at that point, and they got this needle all ready with the stuff in it, and in the middle of a contraction they said, "Do you want it?" And I was not in a position to fight these twenty people all around me, so I said yes. I really, really resent that part. Even now, when I remember my first birth experience, it's like these two different stories happening at one time, the one was this incredible, wonderful, miraculous thing happening, and the other one is just this stupid bureaucratic hassle, just coming out of there feeling really numb. Several years later, a friend of mine was doing research about rape. She was telling me about rape victims, what their psychological state is afterwards. And the kind of numbing that she described, the way they feel about their bodies afterwards, I thought, hey, I know what that feels like, that's how I felt when I came out of the hospital! It's like my body became this thing, all these doctors came and looked at it, and every day you had to lift the blankets and show everybody all your intimate parts. I came out of there feeling like this thing. And at the same time there was this whole other, wonderful, incredible relationship with this baby. I don't think I've got over my anger about that, really, about how much they destroy the beauty of that experience. How they've gotten away with that for so long.

I also felt very ashamed that I had allowed this to happen to me.
Yes, that too. That's part of the helplessness, of feeling if you had been tougher, or smarter or something. I was not very trusting altogether, but I just felt like there wasn't anything to be done. Like, what could I do about it. There just didn't seem to be any alternatives. All the gestures toward independence that I made were met with, you know, they laughed, they just totally denied it all.

Did you have one person that stayed with you from beginning to end though?
Well, my husband, Les, was there. He was very supportive on one level, and very freaked on another level, and therefore not all that helpful. The labour was so short. I remember we tried to play cards. I was far away from home, so I didn't have a lot of family, except my sister who was visiting us at the time. I think one of the reasons I moved back to Winnipeg was to be closer to my family, because I felt very isolated after the baby was born. Before that, as a student, it was nice to get far away from home, and living in downtown Toronto was adventurous. But after I had the baby, it wasn't

a very supportive place to live. I lost most of my social group, because they were graduate students, and my experience was so different from what I'd been doing before. I was very lonely that first year with her. We were living very close to downtown Toronto, and at that time — probably still — having a little baby there was such an unusual thing. Anywhere I went, people would make such a fuss, "Oh, a baby! A real baby! Look at that!" and they'd come and talk to me, and just ooh and aah. When we moved back to Winnipeg, when she was one, I remember you could go anywhere here and people wouldn't even look at your baby. I had to get used to that at first!

The second birth was three years later, and I was a little more prepared about the hospital experience, a little more determined to get what I wanted. But I ended up also having a bad doctor. I was having these kind of contractions, in the last month which are really good to have, because it means you're doing your labour in advance. I was having those quite a lot. So about a week or so before the due date the doctor checked me and he said, "You're already three centimetres dilated." So I thought, oh, that sounds great! Doing all my labour without even knowing it, go in for an hour, that'll be great. And then he said, "So we'll have to induce you." And again, I just wasn't tough enough to fight with him over that.

Why did that mean that he had to induce you?

Well, he said because I was already dilated. Later I found out that that is not a reason to be induced at all. But I went in and was induced. I had a half-hour labour. I had about ten contractions! They were really violent contractions because of the inducement. Les was there again with me, and they sent him out for coffee, and he almost missed the entire thing, because it was so fast. In both of these experiences, actually, they kept saying, oh it'll be hours, it'll be hours, and it was so much shorter than they said. It was really short. And again, I felt powerless. It was different things this time, they didn't give me an epidural, but they did the shaving, and episiotomy and all that stuff. Afterwards you have to walk around with these stitches, for so long, all the pain really afterwards is about those stupid stitches. That was really annoying. I did actually discuss that with him, but there didn't seem to be any way to avoid it at that time. I think now things have changed a bit, you can discuss these things a little more. I also lost a lot of blood, because of how fast it was, and so I had to have a blood transfusion, which was really scary, I was just freaked by that. And then I couldn't leave the hospital because the baby had jaundice. I was all packed and ready to leave, and they said, we'll just have to get the doctor's word on the baby. And then they said, you can't leave, and she had to be under this stupid lamp, so I would walk down the hall and stand in front of the nursery and look at my baby for hours. They all thought I was nuts. And then, yeah, my suitcase was all packed, and they came and said, no, sorry, your baby has to stay another day. You can go home but your baby has to stay. I just sat down and cried, so they said, OK, you can stay too, and I did. It was a horrendous experience, although in some ways it was not as bad as the first birth — well, it was mainly not as bad because I had been through it once already!

When she came home, she didn't gain any weight, and she cried non-stop. I took her to the pediatrician a couple of times, and he said, oh it's just colic. So I tried to be really calm about it, but it was so different than with my first baby, who never cried at all when she was little. I had this feeling all the time that there was something wrong, but the doctor kept saying there was nothing wrong, and you know how it is, you sort of pretend there's nothing wrong. I knew she was in this really formative stage, you know, first few months, learning how to respond to the world. So what I did was, I just talked to her as if she wasn't screaming. I couldn't take her out much, because she was screaming all the time. Finally when she was four months old, I was visiting my mother, and the baby just woke up from her nap, and I was feeding her, and she'd had about two little sucks of milk and she started screaming, and my mother said, "Di, that's no colic, there's no baby that has colic after they just got up from a nap, just barely started feeding." She said, "You go back to the doctor." By then I needed somebody to say that to me. So I went back to the doctor again. Later I found out my doctor was sick and dying of cancer at the time, which may explain why he wasn't more attentive. So he did this little urine test, and she had a bladder infection. Apparently this is quite common in little girls, and he should have easily been able to detect that sooner. He gave us some antibiotics, and two weeks later she turned into this totally different, happy person. She's actually a very happy, upbeat kid. She's a happier kid, really, than the other one, who never had any pain at all, I'm sure, the first year.

So which age did you like best, when they're small babies or a little older?
My favourite time was from when they were born till when they started school, I was just a passionate mother during that time. And after they started going to school, they started having such divided interests, and I did, too. I loved breast-feeding, I loved teaching them, watching them learn how to walk and talk, and language development, that was just fascinating. And play — it recalled for me so much of my own childhood play, and it was like being a little kid again with them, and it was such a lovely excuse to

spend a lot of time in the park, in the wading pool. I was unemployed during some of that time, and part of me was glad. Part of me wished I was earning money, but I had quite a lot of time with them, which I'm very happy for.

Do you think now that hurt them or yourself?
Oh no. It's just that later when they went to school, I did start doing other things, I had to learn how to be more balanced again — no, I mean it was great, it was just a little hard to make the switch again.

Did you have any help at home?
No. For our first baby, my husband, Les, was working very long, late hours. I remember I did try to take a course that year she was born. Les was working an evening shift, starting late afternoon and going till midnight, something like that, got home about one o'clock. I found it really hard to eat during that time. So I would always wait up for him, or I would go to bed, and then I would get up and eat with him, because I couldn't eat alone, when I was pregnant and after. And so this baby had this very weird sleeping pattern. I remember I took this language course at nine o'clock in the morning, because I thought all babies got up early in the morning. And I had this baby that stayed up half the night and slept till noon, so it was like getting up in the middle of the night. It was really bizarre, so I quit.

What else comes to your mind about child raising or childbirth?
Well, something I did find very difficult, I did work full-time from when Lisa was a year old till Ali was born, and I found that really hard. I was just so torn, I found it incredibly hard to leave my baby every day, although it was probably good for us in one way, but it just sort of ripped me up every day. So I'd rush home after, and I didn't give myself enough time in between, to sort of get rested, so I was frazzled a lot. My guilt about leaving her was also really reinforced by my mother and father. All the time I was a student I was supposed to be earning money, and then when I was earning money I was supposed to be at home with my baby. That was really hard. And then when I was pregnant, I found the attitudes of the people where I was working really difficult. I would say that has changed, I mean every woman now works when she has children in one way or another. I still feel that conflict, actually, as a mother, I still find it hard to be self-assertive and independent, a person in the world, and also try to be really nurturing and giving to my children. Sometimes it's a creative tension, a very creative one, but sometimes it's a very problematic one, in terms of energy and so on. I think the model that we had from our own mothers was so very much the one model and

not the other, so that you sort of have to invent this other one. And I think it is getting easier for younger women, in some ways. Sometimes, I must say, I envy my own mother and also my grandmother that way, whose careers were centred on homemaking.

I didn't have a support group when my daughters were born, but then I developed one after that, especially after the second one was born. I had these two young children, and that's when I found all these other young women who had young children, and it was wonderful. That's really when I learned how to be friends with women, I think, which I hadn't known how to do very well before. And spent really a lot of time with them, just lived this sort of strange life of, you know, life with young children, always being immediately ready for whatever is the next thing. I remember it as a time of people dropping by all the time, people in and out all the time, and having to make these huge meals and be ready for all these unexpected things. I think it was a wonderful thing for me to go through, but I would say it's not really me. I think, naturally, I like to be alone more, I like to do more silent things, you know. But it was sort of a nice thing to do for a few years, to be so external, and so social.

Did you go out to meet other women with children for the sake of your children mostly, or for your own sake?

Oh no, for my own sake. I was intellectually desperately lonely during that time. I just loved doing all this stuff with the children, I even took some early childhood courses. I was really into that, but at the same time there was this other part of me, the part of me that thinks and needs to talk. I remember people would come to my house and I would just corner them and start going on and on and on about a book I'd read or some idea that was in my head, and most of them were eying the door and trying to see when they could get away, I think. Some of them felt a little trapped by this desperate need of mine for conversation. I think my writing came out of that, partly, this desperate need for an audience, you know, and not having it there. With writing, you invent an audience in your head and you write it down for them, right. And then finding a real one out there, that was neat.

I got married in '71, and we had this naïve idea that we were going to revise all the roles. From the beginning we thought that we wouldn't have these inherited roles, we would just play around with them and change them the way we wanted. We found it's not nearly as easy to do that as you think. First of all, there's all the things inside you, the structure, whether you want it or not, and also just the way the rest of the world is set up. It's not possible for you to change everything as quickly as you want to. I remember that as being a really frustrating thing for me. My father was very controlling in the family in some ways, but he was proud of being the provider. For my husband, being the provider was not valuable in itself. It didn't have the worth that it did previously, because of the fact that I and other women were saying that we don't want to be totally dependent. This has been a very confusing thing, trying to change all that, around children and everything.

Because somebody still has to look after the children.
You can't just divide it up and say, you'll do half and half. I did find I had this incredible fund of knowledge about children inside me that I didn't even know I had, from my own mother, which he doesn't have. And also all these other young women that I knew, I did manage to find this wonderful support group and everything, and he didn't have that. And then also, I didn't know how terribly much — I guess young parents never know this — how terribly much energy and time it's going to take, those children, and how totally your life is going to change because of them. When I went back to school to do my Ph.D., I felt so much more grounded and centred than I had before, and more clear-thinking, but at the same time the time factor and the energy factor was so limited.

What about your knowledge of the physical aspects of pregnancy, birth, and so on, did you know enough about it, or had you read enough, did you find the reading material you wanted?
Well, like I said, I felt that I didn't know anything about it when I became pregnant, and then because I was a graduate student, of course, I went and got all the books I could find about pregnancy and childbirth and childrearing and stuff. I think I read far too much. I knew all the things that could go wrong, and all the things you should do, and all the things you shouldn't do, and all the details of children's development; too much stuff, and thought about it too much. What would have been more helpful is to have a community, a women's community, to be part of. I think the whole experience of becoming a mother revised my approach to the world in a very radical way. After that it became much more listening to my own mother, and recognizing the need for continuity with my past, and just learning how to approach the world through my experience of it, my physical and also my emotional experience of it, rather than what you read in a book.

Was it ever a thought in your mind not to have children?
I didn't plan my life very — what's the right way to say this? When I finished high school, I didn't have a clear career in mind, but looking

back, I realize I did all the necessary things to make it possible for me to become a writer eventually. I didn't know that at the time, I sort of did that intuitively. It was a very complicated route to get there, but — as far as planning to have them or not planning to have them, it just suddenly seemed like the right thing to do, so we did, and I would have had lots more if we'd had more money. Because I loved it, really. I don't want to imagine not having had any. Because they were so significant for me in becoming a grounded person.

Marjorie Neufeld Martin

Marjorie Neufeld Martin was born Marjorie Anderson in 1944 in Libau, Manitoba. She was married to Jim Neufeld and they had three children, one of whom died in childhood. After Jim's death Marjorie married Gary Martin, with whose two daughters they have four children. Marjorie is an instructor in communications at the University of Manitoba and has a Ph.D. in English literature.

Marjorie Neufeld Martin came to my house for the interview. We sat at the dining-room table, and before we knew it the tape needed to be turned. Her interview covers a variety of parenting experiences: adoption, the chronic illness and death of a child, a subsequent adoption, and the birth by Caesarean section of a third child. Marjorie's morning interview was powerful; she spoke so eloquently about her feelings that the images of her energy and strength lingered with me all day. Not many women can talk so freely about their feelings, and I thank her for the rare gift of sharing her story.

Marjorie, can you tell me about your experiences with motherhood?
Well, my first experience with motherhood was through adoption. My first marriage was to Jim Neufeld, whose parents belonged to the Mennonite community. When we discovered that we would have difficulty having biological children, we decided to adopt. We were too eager to have children to wait and see exactly what our chances were to have biological children.

At that time adoption was very, very easy. We waited about two months — now I think it's seven years. I taught right up until June — we had applied at the end of May — and we picked up our first daughter on the 12th of July. So it was a very quick process. And when I think back to my first introduction to motherhood, I look upon it as the first miracle of my life. It was a wonderful experience, and subsequently I had the experience of giving birth to a child. I don't think I could rate one above the other. I am so pleased that I had both experiences, because they were both equally joyous. When we went to pick up our child, we picked her up at the hospital; at that time they allowed you to go right to the hospital. The birth mother had already gone home, so there was no chance of meeting. Our child, whom we named Pamela Dawn, was fourteen days old when we picked her up. I still remember walking past the nursery window, and a nurse had this pretty little baby in her arms. I thought, What a lovely baby! and then I realized that this was our baby. I remember that flood of joy and excitement that never really left. And I can't think of any way that this feeling was much different from the flood of joy I had when I saw the child whom I gave birth to. — So that was our first experience, and I remember it as a time of being "in love" with our child, and I think of it as our first miracle. Then we had other miracles. But there's something profound about that first experience. She was a delightful baby. She learned very quickly, and grew into a happy, lovely little child. And I think, as all first parents, we assumed that she was as wonderful and quick and bright as she was because we were wonderful parents, you see.

Just before her second birthday — we had already applied to adopt a second child, and we were waiting for that — Pamela developed symptoms that were worrisome, and we had to take her to the hospital. We discovered that she had an inoperable brain tumour, and that she would not live more than six months. At that point we had been going through adoption procedures. When our social worker, who had become a friend of ours, had to report that our child was terminally ill, she was told that she couldn't place another child in our home without consent from a committee. The committee that reviewed our case declared that we couldn't adopt; they felt that ours were not the kind of circumstances that a child should go into. The second impulse, after the horror and shock of being told that our child was terminally ill, was that we must have more children. I don't think it was a rational response, it was an emotional one that washed over me. I knew that the decision the committee had made was not the right one for me or for our family. But it was very difficult to know what to do about it.

Our social worker was certainly very sympathetic, and we talked to her about what we should do. We decided to appeal the decision. I sat down and wrote a long letter. I invited the committee to come into our home and talk to us and to our friends, and then make a decision, but not to make a decision without knowing us. Friends of ours who lived in the neighbourhood and some others who also felt very strongly, wrote letters and made phone calls to Children's Aid. At that time, my mother moved in with us. (She stayed for seven years after that.) She was a widow who had been living in an apartment on her own, and she moved in with the idea that she would help us care for Pamela. After this the Children's Aid changed their decision, they decided they would place a child with us. One of the factors that made them feel comfortable about it was that my mother was going to live with us. And in looking back, I realize that that they were wise, because it would have been very difficult for us to care for our new daughter, Heidi, in the way that she needed to be cared for if we hadn't had my mother's help, because at that time Pamela was in a great deal of pain, and she would sometimes be up all night.

When Heidi came, we worked out a system. I would sleep one night and my husband would sleep the other night, and we would take turns being up with our sick child. My mother looked after Heidi at night when she woke up for her bottle. Consequently, there has been a bonding between my mother and Heidi that is very evident even today. My mother has twenty-four grandchildren now, but there's something special about Heidi, and I think that, really, Heidi grew up with three parents — my mom, her dad, and me.

We didn't have the experience of picking Heidi up at the hospital; we went to Children's Aid, and they brought her into a room in a little crib. She was twelve days old. It was a different experience from picking up Pamela at the hospital. In my experience of adopting children, the only sadness that I had was that I hadn't had some part in creating them, so I wanted to get them as soon as I could. I still remember the joy, the miracle of this little baby that was ours. And I don't have any memories other than one of instant bonding. Certainly that was my experience, and my husband's, too, for he was a natural with children.

Heidi became our light into the future, and I realize now what a tremendous responsibility was put on the head of this little baby, because she became our only child who was able to give us feedback on our parenting. About six months after Pamela was diagnosed, she essentially lost consciousness and became semi-comatose, and this was the state that she lived in for five and a half years. We cared for her at home for five of those years. She needed to be tube-fed and suctioned, because in lying prone, she would gather a lot of fluids, and the possibility of her choking was great.

Heidi was an excellent baby. She seemed to have an innate sense that she needed to allow us to administer to Pamela first. I remember when she was about two, I would be reading to her, and she would hear Pamela call, and would say, you have to go to Pamela! or run to Pamela! or whatever she could say at the time. So she grew up with the sense of caring for others before herself, which I think is a unique quality in Heidi even today.

We had once again applied for adoption, for we wanted more children. Both my husband and I could not get over our delight in girls, so we had applied again for a baby girl. And then I discovered that I was pregnant. We hadn't been told that it was impossible for us to have children, but that there were some difficulties that we just didn't seem to be able to remedy. Then we had to make a decision: should we tell our social worker? What should we do about the baby we were planning to adopt? The only experience we'd had was of adopting children, and we knew how joyous that was. We felt that there was a baby out there who belonged to us, and to say no to this adoption was like handing our child over to someone else. So that was difficult, it really was.

We waited until I was five months pregnant before we told our social worker that we were expecting. She promised that she wouldn't take our name off the list because at that time there was a longer waiting period, and we didn't want our name taken off the list until the child I was carrying was born. And I remember — or maybe it was before we told her — we got a phone call from our social worker, and she asked if we would be prepared to take a child who wasn't born yet, but whose birth parents had indicated that they wanted a very specific background, and our social worker felt that we suited their criteria. It was in summertime and we were at the beach when we got this phone call, and I remember walking along the beach with Jim, thinking, How can we give up this baby who could be ours? But then we also recognized that we had a sick child, we had a toddler, and then there would be another new baby in November, and so we would not be fair to that other baby. I felt in a way that I had the experience of giving up a child, and it made me feel even closer to the women who had given birth to my adopted children, although I had always had a very warm feeling towards those women. Their sorrow and their very wise decisions brought a lot of joy to our lives. Having that sense of giving up a child because it would be best for the child gave me extra empathy with the birth parents.

So then my next experience was my giving birth to a child. I come from a family of eight children, so my mother had certainly had a lot of birthing experience. I was really afraid, and I guess because our oldest daughter was at that time brain-damaged, I had such a terrible fear that something would be wrong with the baby. My mom was still living with us then, and I used to say to her, "Tell me again, Mom, how did you give birth to all these children?" I remember her response would be, "Marjorie, it's just natural. It's just natural." She had had all eight of us at home. She said that the first one was frightening; she had decided that she would have it by natural childbirth, but when the pains became too strong, she said she just asked for relief. But after that one, it seemed that the rest of us just came, and she didn't have any stories of anxiety or fear or anything like that. I also talked with my aunt, who had had seven children. I was almost obsessed with talking about how women lived through giving birth. And my aunt's response was, "Well, the first batch . . . the second batch . . ." [laughs] and I thought, If somebody could sit here, look alive and healthy, and talk about "batches" of children, then surely I could give birth to this first one. We did join a Lamaze group, because I wanted to give birth to my child naturally. I remember a tour of the Health Sciences Centre, the labour and delivery floor, which was rather daunting. I never really got over the fear of giving birth.

Did you talk to your doctor about it at all?

No, but I talked a lot to my family. I guess I've always done that. I have such a large, receptive family that I could talk to them about anything.

I was not conscious during the actual experience of giving birth to our daughter. There is some sadness in that for me. We had requested that I have an epidural and be awake for the delivery and that my husband be present for the birth. Both requests were denied. One because the anesthesiologist on duty was only experienced with general anesthetic and the other because, at that time [1976], fathers weren't allowed in during a Caesarean section. I remember feeling a sadness for Jim because he wanted to be part of the experience. I remember the morning of our daughter's birth. The nurses had "prepped" me — the night before I had to suffer the indignity of having my stomach swabbed with iodine and shaved — and they put me on a stretcher to take me to the operating room. Jim had to stay behind in the hall, and I watched him standing there alone as they wheeled me away. I'm glad that fathers are allowed in now. They should be.

When they got me to the operating room, the staff wasn't ready, so I had to stay outside in the corridor for a short time — an eternity at that time. I remember shivering with cold or fear and saying to the doctor when he arrived, "I've changed my mind. I'm not going to have this baby." He humoured me by laughing, but then declared everything ready, so I was wheeled into the operating room. They used pentothol to put me under, and I saw them drop the drug into my I.V. The last thing I saw, literally, was the surgeon with the knife, the scalpel raised, because with a Caesarean section, they have just two minutes to get to the baby before the anesthetic gets into the baby's system. It's an extremely bloody operation, because they don't have time to clamp any vessels, so they slash, I think, literally. And what they removed from me was a healthy baby girl.

When I came out of the anesthetic I just remember this floating sensation. It seemed like I was floating on a cloud, and voices were coming from somewhere. Faces would appear, and I was in and out of consciousness. The first words I remember about our child was that they said, "Mrs. Neufeld, you have a *healthy* baby girl." Which I really appreciated, because I think they knew our story. And then I remember a flood of the same kind of wonder and excitement. With every face that appeared, I leapt up and kissed it! Apparently there was a nurse, there was a doctor, my sister-in-law who worked at the hospital, I leapt up and kissed them all and promised them my life and all my treasures. I was just totally drunk with joy for about two days after that. I have a letter that I wrote to a cousin who was overseas at the time, and she brought it to me not too long ago. I read it, and it's like it was written by somebody high on something, because I couldn't get out enough superlatives for the experience. So I really am thankful for how it turned out. My husband was too. It was a joy that was accentuated by tremendous relief that the child was healthy, and by the recognition of our good fortune.

When you have a Caesarean, you of course aren't allowed to get out of bed the first day, and the baby goes into an incubator. So usually you don't see the baby for a day. But my doctor — I thank him very much for this — had said to the nurses that he thought that I would not be able to stay in that bed if I didn't get a sight of this baby. So they wheeled me on the stretcher into the nursery. I was still a bit groggy from the anesthetic when they showed me our baby, and I remember being amazed at seeing this tiny, tiny little girl. I guess because my husband was very dark and muscular, I anticipated a large male child. But there was this tiny, little, blonde baby girl. Also I remember seeing a hairy little bum, because she was on her stomach with her legs drawn up, and a broad nose. The Neufelds have very broad noses, and I remember thinking, Ah, she has a Neufeld nose! I don't know where the hairy bum came from! It was excellent that I did see her, because I really would have found it difficult that first day. My husband kept running back and forth to the nursery, and I'd ask, "Well what's she like?" and he'd say, "Oh, she's beautiful, just beautiful!" Or I'd say, "Well what are her fingers like?" "They're beautiful!" "What are her toes like?" "They're beautiful!" He obviously had the same feeling and experience that I did.

I stayed in the hospital eight days. The third day after the birth was very painful, because that's when gas pains from having abdominal surgery set in. I never experienced a labour pain with any of the children. I like to say that I've had all sorts of children but never a labour pain! But those were painful. So I feel that I experienced some of the pain of childbirth. And the experience in the hospital was just a supremely joyous one. The nurses were tremendous, everything went well, and the baby was healthy. Also, I had my first experience of nursing, which I had missed with adoption. I remember holding Pamela and Heidi, and yearning to be able to nurse them. I really enjoyed the experience of nursing, and I nursed Renata for eight months, and then had to stop, because we went away for a weekend. The milk had dried up by the time I came back. I just never could get started again. So nursing was a unique part of that birth experience.

Can you talk about how the experience of adoption and of giving birth were similar?

Yes, when I saw our daughter Renata in the nursery that first time, it was a very similar experience to when I saw Heidi and Pamela the first time. And perhaps one contributing factor was that I was not conscious when giving birth to her, so the experiences seemed very similar. Or perhaps it's because of my nature. If somebody gave me a child to care for, no matter where or how the child came, I would just instantly do it. I often think that the feelings I had when I first saw Renata, first saw Heidi, first saw Pamela, were very similar. I just remember the tremendous sense of awe and joy. I'd like to be an advocate for adoption, for people who suffer a lot of agony if they can't give birth to a child. The joy that you have can be different in some ways, but it's equally wonderful. And I would really like people to know that, because that's been my experience.

You've had an awful lot of pain in your life, and it seems to me that you learned something from each of these experiences, painful as they are.

Well, certainly when I look back to the joys and pain of my life, I realize that from the pain I have become conscious in a way that I couldn't have without it — conscious of the joys of motherhood, the joys of life, of the brevity and tenuousness of life. One thing I remember about my feelings when caring for our child who was going to die, was, how can you watch your child die? Everything inside of us, all instincts are to care for and protect our children, and to nurture and to see them grow. I have a cousin who is extremely important in my life, and I remember saying to her, "Dawn, how can I watch my child die?" and she said, "Don't. Watch her live." And that's what I did, for five and a half years. And there were days and nights when we had a lot of agony, when, before she lost consciousness, she was in pain, and would just scream and scream, and we couldn't do anything. She'd say, "My head is hurting, help me, help me!" and we couldn't. The agony of that! But at the end of the day, when I wondered how we would get through the next day, I just thought, She's still alive, and we can still care for her and love her. It kept me going all those years, and it was something that I used again when my husband got ill and died. I watched him live, and I watched our daughter live.

Pamela died when she was seven and a half. At the time, our other girls were five and two. I remember after she died hearing mothers complain about their children, and feeling horrified. How could they ever complain! It took me a long time to get over the sense that I was doing a terrible thing if I ever felt weary with my children. I never allowed myself that feeling. I can now. Sometimes now I even say to my husband, "Ugh, let's go away for two days!" and I can accept that, but for a long time I couldn't, because no matter what was going on, they were alive and they were healthy. This has helped me over the years. When I have the "ordinary" agonies of parenting children — disappointments, frustrations, or anger — I always come back to the thought that, no matter what, I am so happy that they are alive and well.

What I would like to talk about to complete my experience of having children is my experience of having stepchildren. My first husband became ill and was diagnosed with cancer of the prostate just four years after Pamela died. It was of course a tremendous blow, and the same sense of incredulousness that we had when we discovered Pamela was ill. Once again, I thought very much about watching him live, and he did live, with as much joy as anyone I've ever seen, until the end. He taught us all a lot.

Two years later, when I married Gary, I acquired two more daughters, Cheryl and Dena. My fear with being a stepmother is that I won't be able to give my stepchildren the distance that they may want or need. I don't have any difficulty in thinking of them as children of mine. I don't have any difficulty in accepting that they had a mother, who mothered them well for many years; but I've just incorporated them into my heart, and I worry about them, agonize about them, take pride and joy in them as I do Heidi and Renata. It has been a joyous experience of parenting. I would not want to do without any of these experiences, and I'm trying to think, Are there any others that I haven't had? [laughs] I am fortunate in that I've gained two more exceptional children. Gary and I have talked about this experience. When you're a stepparent, you have a sense of responsibility and caring for your spouse, who is their natural parent, for the children, because you take them in and care for them. But I think above and beyond that you also have a sense of doing something that their other natural parent couldn't do. I have some sense of the agony that Cheryl and Dena's mother must have gone through in dying and leaving her children before she could see them grown. I know the agony Jim went through in dying and leaving his children. And I feel that in a way Gary and I are doing something for these people, for our children's other two parents.

Mrs. A

Mrs. A, who asked that her name not be used, was born in 1912. She moved to Mexico with her parents and later returned to Manitoba to live. She and her husband had fourteen children, of whom ten survived to adulthood. She has some astute observations on breast-feeding.

Between 1922 and 1927, several thousand Mennonites belonging to the two most conservative groups that had come to Canada from Ukraine in the 1870s immigrated to Mexico. They left Canada in protest of the secularization process that required that they conduct their schools in the English language. In the late 1950s a number of these Mennonite families returned to Canada to escape a severe drought in Mexico. The poorest of these returning immigrants became migrant agricultural workers. Mrs A. was part of this immigration back to Canada.

[Translated from Plautdietsch]

Where were you born, and how big was your family?
I was born in Manitoba, not far from Haskett. I am the youngest in the family. My sisters were much older, they had left home by then. Then in 1922 my parents moved to Mexico. I was ten years old at the time. So I attended school in Mexico as well. And when I thought I was grown up —

When was that, when you thought you were grown up?
Well, I was seventeen by that time, and already getting married. People thought that was much too young. But my parents were old, they were no longer young, and so I said to them, "Why shouldn't I get married if I have the chance? you're already old, and if you're suddenly gone, I'll be alone." And so we got married, and of course we got to work, we wanted to farm. But in those first years in Mexico, people didn't quite know what would grow there, all there was was corn and beans. There was no grain at the time. They did a lot of experimenting with oats and other things, but it got much better later on. At first the wheat didn't really take. But they discovered different varieties of oats, and some did better than others, especially years later, with the irrigation systems. But in those years, when we were young, times were hard in Mexico. Many babies died, too. People didn't know how to feed their children. They were poor and didn't know better, and so many children died. They couldn't digest cow's milk, and there was no other kind of milk. So it had to be very diluted, and that's what they gave the children, they were not able to breast-feed. And the cows' milk was much too strong for the children, and baby food like there is now was not available then. Many of them got diarrhea, and had to die of diarrhea. Then things progressed further and further, and they got in more of the kinds of things to help children grow.

Did any of your children die?
Not as babies. Well, we had one that died of whooping cough, who lived for only fifteen days. And then we buried some at an older age. But they had other illnesses. Some of our children were very sick at times, but they were never sickly, like many others. I breast-fed most of them. And so then it wasn't so bad.

And where were your children born, at home or in the hospital?
No, just at home, with the women. A lot of young women also died because they had only their husbands to look after them. It was different there at that time, the doctor couldn't take them, and so they had to die with their baby. That happened a lot. In later years that improved; in later years they would also go to the hospital, but not when we were young.

Was it always a woman you knew?
Yes, it was always one of our people. It happened the odd time that a doctor would come, if the woman couldn't manage, a doctor would come from Cusi [Mexico], I think he was English. It would finally get to that point, if she was dying, he would have to come. But many simply had to die of it.

What was the reason, why did they die?
It just couldn't be born.

The baby would be too big, or turned the wrong way, or —
Yes, like that. And the women [who acted as midwives] weren't well enough educated. Yes, there was a lot of that. But things kept improving. Even so, there was a time in later years, when it was so very dry, times were hard, in the forties; times were very hard in the forties.

When a woman found out she was pregnant again, did she tell anyone about it or not?
No. They didn't go to the doctor the way they do here. No, they just waited until it was time, and then the midwife had to be fetched. And they did everything they could there, they could do a lot, but there was also a lot they weren't able to do.

And the children didn't know anything about it either, did they?
No, they weren't told, like nowadays. That was considered very bad, if the children asked about it, they were hushed up quickly, they weren't supposed to. [laughs] But there were always children who knew very well what was going on. They had to go to the neighbours' when a baby was born. Overnight too, however it happened. But once they came home again there would be a new baby. And the children knew that too, then, that was fine and good.

Do you find it strange now, to hear your children tell their children?
In a way no, but I think it can be overdone, too. The children don't need to be reminded of it all the time. But neither should one say, "Be quiet and shame on you, you don't need to know that." That shouldn't be said either. They could be told, "You're going to have another brother or sister." Nowadays everything is explained to children in detail, I think it shouldn't be necessary. But when we were living here in Canada again, we would occasionally read the *Winnipeg Free Press*. Well, I wasn't able to read it, but those who could, did. And there were women who would write in and say the children were so curious. They knew something, but the one woman said, her children would ask questions, too, much more than one would answer. And so the child had asked where the baby was, and she had answered, "It comes from a place close to my heart." And that had satisfied the child.

When women had large families, were they happy or not?
Some were happy, some were not happy. Because usually the large families

were the poorest. They were so very poor, and so they would be looked at sideways: yes, they had children, but weren't able to feed them. That was really a pity. We didn't know that there was something we could do about it. We believed this was how God had ordained it, it had to be like that. Some had few and some had many, but generally families were quite large.

None of your children died at birth?
No, they were all born safely, none of them died at birth. Our first one was born with a harelip, and I couldn't breast-feed him properly; his palate was open as well as his lip. He was a very sickly baby because I couldn't feed him properly. He died at three months. The next one was a very healthy baby, he lived. The third one lived till he was six years old, he was a bit of a sickly child, too, but he made it to school age, and then he got a disease, a respiratory infection. And he died of that, he was very ill. And later we had another child like that. But in between I had three more children, and one of those lived to age two and a half. She was otherwise healthy, a very beautiful little girl, but she also got that sickness. They could swallow, but they couldn't breathe. They had great difficulty breathing. It was just in the air. And so she had to die, too. And none of the others died, they all grew to adulthood.

It must have been very hard to bury your children. Can you imagine your life without children? They are a big part of life, aren't they.
Oh, yes. Yes, yes, very much so. I would have been very sorry if I hadn't been able to have children.

How old were you when you had your first child?
Just over eighteen. Yes, I was young. But I was able to breast-feed the first few, so there was some space between them, about two years; then we'd think that was manageable. There were some parents who had a baby every year, and sometimes two at a time.

Well, doctors are saying now that breast-feeding is much healthier.
Yes, now the doctors are for it, but in the beginning, the first years we were here [in Canada], they would say, if you don't want to, just don't start. But now they're saying something else. I think that God created it that way. And now there are also those who believe they can't do it. But they say that really, unless the woman is very unhealthy, there is no such thing, it's all in the head. If they just persisted — but these days they seem to be embarrassed.

They are embarrassed or they think they don't have the time or whatever.
No. They don't have time, or they have jobs, and then they don't start with

it — it's really too bad, the child is much healthier if the mother breast-feeds it. One of my daughters, the second-youngest, with her first child thought too that was impossible. I told her, "That's just in your head that you can't do it." "No," she said, and I didn't know that, but it was true, she really wasn't able to. But she was able to breast-feed all her other children. Now she doesn't believe herself that it was impossible.They now have four children. I also have some children who are not able to have children. But there are enough! My oldest daughter has many children, and she already has as many grandchildren as I have.

I wanted to ask you about your moves. How was the journey from Mexico to Canada?

Oh we had an interesting — [laughs] I've sometimes said, you could write a book about it. We moved back to Canada in 1954, I think I must have been forty-three. We were a huge group of poor people who wanted to earn some money. And there was a Peter Fehr, he had been in Canada for quite some time already, he came to Mexico, and we drove with him. Five families in one of those big trucks. We had built a bench for each family in the back, and that's where we sat! [laughs]

Out in the open! Or did you have a roof?

There was a tent over top, with a bit of open space between the truck box and the tent. That was in May. And the man would always drive around the cities, he wouldn't drive through them, and once in a while we would come to a water puddle, where the women would wash their diapers. But I was fortunate, all my children were old enough to be out of diapers. My youngest was two years old. Well, he may have needed a diaper once in a while, but mostly not; the other women had younger children. But we were five families; one family had five children, the others each had seven children, all in one truck! [laughs]

The men sat in front?

No.The families sat together. Yes, there were all kinds of things. This man — we didn't know this of course, we weren't familiar with everything, when he brought us here to Canada, none of us spoke any English, and he said he would give us jobs. As it turned out he had no work to offer us.

He came from Canada, this Peter Fehr?

Yes. Although originally he was from Mexico. Yes, and so we needed enough for the trip — we had brought food with us, but we had no money to pay the trip with, we had to earn it here. When we first arrived here, he didn't even have a house. So we slept outdoors, and the first night it rained, and it was cold. After the rain it froze, outside under the open sky. Eventually he found a house, but he didn't tell us who had lived there before. We found out later that he had been living there, and that they didn't really want him there any more. It was an old brick house, a big two-storey house, but because he had so many people with him, they allowed it. So then all five families lived together in that one house. And with all those five families, there were quite some squabbles! [laughs]

Yes, I can imagine! What would they be about?
Well, between the children, there were a lot of disagreements, people would complain a lot. Eventually the men got jobs along with the children who were old enough to work too, weeding beets. Fehr would drive them, we didn't have vehicles, of course, and they would weed beets and could then pay off the trip.

And finally, did you all stay together or did you go your separate ways?
No, there were other people, word got around that we were so poor, and then from elsewhere, the Old Mennonites from Kitchener, they would sometimes bring all kinds of things for us, and food, too, one time they brought us things from Vineland, and finally we were able to move apart, although some of us, we and two other families, we lived together in a house for a while after that yet, too, in an old house, there was enough room for all of us. And then we kept going, and once we were able to move on again they helped us out too, these were the ones from Russia. And then our family worked on a peach farm. They had sixty acres of peach trees. So that first year we worked on the peach farm. But then we thought, In the winter there will be no more work here, and so we went to B.C., northern B.C., in the bush. So our family worked at the sawmill in the bush. But they weren't satisfied with the life there, they wanted to go back to Ontario. Well, so we went back again by train. And since then we have always worked in Ontario. Yes, and eventually we earned enough to help ourselves. And then all the Mennonite people wanted a place where they could live together and have their own church. So they found this place near Rainy River [Ontario], and each of us got a piece of land there, so that we could be independent. But for people who didn't have the necessary big machinery the land wasn't really workable. And we found out later that there was much less rainfall there. It's called "Rainy River," and there was a fair bit of rain, but it would come all at once, either in spring or in fall. It would be too wet. It was very difficult there. Yes, we never got very far ahead.

What kind of work did you enjoy most?

I think I enjoyed all of it. I would often say, a housewife's lot is like a wheel of infinity. It was always from morning to night you had your work, and the next morning it was the same thing all over again. And it was never visible.

Did you enjoy looking after the children?

Oh yes! I very much enjoyed looking after the children. I always tried not to neglect them. And I never had babysitters. I was at home with the children. Well, I did have kitchen help at times, when the children were small. Once our oldest children were old enough to help, they did. That was something my husband made sure of. They had to help. It wasn't like it is now. Nowadays children don't have to do anything at home. They have their own things, toys. But they don't need to help their mother with the dishes. In those days the oldest girls, as soon as they were able, had to wash dishes. Washing dishes was girls' work. And that's not the way it is now. They don't do it, they prefer to go out with their friends, and let their mothers do it by themselves.

Susanna Edith Klassen

Susanna Edith (Klassen) Klassen, my younger sister, was born in 1938 in Winnipeg. She and her husband, John, now divorced, have three children. Susanna was a psychiatric nurse and part-time student at York University at the time of the interview. She and her husband moved to Toronto in 1961 and were there when our first baby was born and died in 1962. Four months later she had a baby. It was a painful time for me. I wanted to be supportive of her but I don't think I was. When we talked about her birth giving twenty-six years later in my living room, I was hearing some of her story for the first time. She had experienced both sides of the hospital — as a nurse and as a patient/expectant mother.

I BECAME PREGNANT with Jonathan a year after I got married, and I remember at the time I was becoming restless about my work and thinking of going into pediatrics. I was starting to apply to the Sick Children's Hospital when I discovered that I was expecting a baby myself. I was very excited. When I went to work after I found that I was expecting a baby, I was so elated I couldn't hold it back, and I told everyone. It wasn't as though I had been longing to have a baby, but when it happened, it was the best thing that had ever happened to me. I remember also doing a lot of reading about parenthood, and about the importance of nurturing the infant, and that helped me to become very aware of my maternal instincts and my wish to nurture the child. I also became aware that there were many things in society that did not confirm this, especially the way we gave birth and the way the mother was allowed to care for the baby after birth. Early in my pregnancy I read an article about rooming-in. I had been working in maternity, so I had seen the way women gave birth and the way they cared for their babies, and the four-hour feeding, and letting babies cry. I always thought there was something not quite right about that. I talked to my obstetrician about having rooming-in in the hospital when my baby was born, and he learned that this was against the hospital's policy. So I went and looked for another doctor who worked at a hospital where I could have rooming-in, even though by today's standards it was not really rooming-in. I had the baby all day and all night, because I asked for it, but I wasn't able to have him until two or three days after I had given birth. With Jonathan the labour was induced, and when I think back now I think it was induced because the doctor wanted to go on a skiing trip. I don't think I could really believe that at the time, because I wouldn't have wanted to think that he might do something like that.

What reasons did he give?

There was a valid reason for me going into hospital, because I'd had something, that I guess was false labour, or considered false labour, a couple of nights before, and when I went to see him I was already three days overdue and I was dilated, so he wanted to admit me.

What was it like to be induced?

Well, all they did was break the water. They didn't give me Pitocin. My labours were all kind of uneventful, especially with Jonathan and Joel, they were both four hours. I guess I thought of them as being very painful, I remember saying to my doctor at one time that he hadn't really known what he was talking about when he said that it wouldn't be all that painful. I couldn't have my husband there during the first two, but insisted, on the third one.

What about anesthesia?

Well, I did have the spinal, or epidurals. I quite frankly can't remember whether I had Demerol. I don't think I did, but the third one stands out in my memory, because she was in a different position, and it was very very painful labour, I couldn't quite imagine how anything could be so painful. She was born with her face up, rather than her face down. And I guess the back of the head pressing against the backbone was what caused such pain.

But what I remember is that after the births I was always in a very elated state, and I just loved it, I loved nurturing and breast-feeding. I always think now that if I hadn't been able to breast-feed, that would have been very sad and very tragic. And sometimes I wonder why I don't have stronger feelings about the fact that I didn't give birth to my children naturally, whether it's something that I'm not in touch with, or because I had such a satisfying experience with them after the birth.

Do you know why you felt so strongly about breast-feeding and rooming-in?
When I think of reading about infant care and the bonding, some of the things that I read were already pointing to what we now know about the importance of the bonding. Because I know that I used to have very strong maternal feelings towards them when I was carrying them, and certainly they became much stronger after I had them, and I just felt it was the best thing for them. I remember with Jonathan I had very sore nipples, and I called my doctor one time, and she said, well do you want to give up breast-feeding? I couldn't believe that she had even said it. Of course, it strengthened my determination to continue.

How did you solve the problem then?
I would walk around the apartment with my nipples uncovered and I'd use a heat lamp. And I'd use lanolin cream. I became aware of La Leche League when I was nursing Joel, when I was having some problems, because he was one of these babies that refused to conform to the four-hour schedule. Jonathan more or less conformed to it; he would have his periods when he would want it more often. He would also have periods when he would sleep for a long, long time, and Joel absolutely refused to do any of that, he insisted on every two hours. And so I was at the point where I was worried that there was something wrong or that he wasn't getting enough food, and I remember calling my doctor one day and I had been talking to him quite often about the problem and at that time he said to me, "Well don't you think it's about time to give up?"

How old was he then?
Joel? He must have been three or four months old. And that same night I was looking at the paper, and I came across an announcement about La Leche League. I think I had actually been reading the La Leche book, but somehow it wasn't enough. I needed some kind of personal support, and so I picked up the phone immediately and started going to some of the meetings, and actually became quite involved in La Leche League. I managed to nurse Joel until he was eleven months old. I had many discussions with my doctor about how disappointed I was about the medical profession and

their ignorance about breast-feeding. I think that the urge was very, very strong, the maternal urge was very strong, that's the way I experienced it, anyway. I still look back at it as one of the best times of my life, a very satisfying experience, to breast-feed.

In what other ways did your professional nursing experience influence you, do you think?
I guess the most important experience I had there isn't related to breast-feeding necessarily, but I remember working in pediatrics, and we had a premature baby on the ward. We used to pick up this baby a lot, he was sort of the pet of the floor, and everybody picked him up and cuddled him. And then one day the head nurse decided that this baby was becoming spoiled, and she gave us orders not to pick him up. And to me it just did not seem right. I didn't have anything to go by to refute her decision, but it didn't seem right, I didn't think that we could spoil a baby, and I thought it was very cruel to let him cry. That really left a mark on my memory, about how infants should be cared for, and somehow I've always felt that babies couldn't be spoiled by picking them up. I did struggle with that a lot with my first and my second, though. Especially with Joel, when he was always crying every two hours. Then I thought, Well, maybe there is some truth to this. But after my experience with La Leche League, I became more and more convinced that you couldn't spoil babies.

Did you find other women with babies that wanted to be picked up and fed every two hours, too?
In La Leche League? Oh yes, the attitude there was entirely different. You just picked up the baby and fed it when it was crying, if it was hungry. If babies aren't hungry, they'll let you know. And also the whole idea that they need sucking, not necessarily food all the time, but they need the sucking, and that that's an important need, it's not something they should be deprived of.

What about prenatal care, did you feel that the doctor took the time to talk to you about anything you wanted to talk about?
I don't think I ever felt terribly free to talk to doctors, and probably because I was a nurse I had this idea that I didn't want to look foolish. I had three healthy pregnancies, in fact I think I was probably healthier when I was pregnant than when I wasn't. When I look at the kind of prenatal classes they have now and the Lamaze and all that, if I could have had some of that, I would have been much better off.

There used to be a lot of emphasis on weight gain. Was there a certain weight gain that you were not supposed to exceed?

Oh yes. I was not supposed to exceed twenty pounds, and I remember one time towards the end of one of the pregnancies, I went in and I had gained a bit more than he thought I should, and he told me I was eating too many peanut butter sandwiches. I worked until November, I believe, and I had Jonathan end of December, and after I quit working, I spent many hours sewing little gowns and things for him, and I made myself a uniform that I always liked, I felt very good in. I've always liked clothes, so I liked maternity clothes as well. I always felt enhanced by my pregnancies. Some women say they can't understand how a pregnant woman can be attractive, but I never felt that it took away from my attractiveness. But the interesting thing is that I also don't have any pictures of myself when I'm pregnant. I have some pictures that were taken at a shower, but I don't have any pictures taken in my own home.

What do you remember about labour?

The pressure to be a good patient was certainly felt. After having worked in obstetrics, I had an idea of what kind of a patient I wanted to be. [laughs] I didn't want nurses to be speaking about me as "that woman over there." [laughs] I wasn't the same though when it came to having rooming-in and having the baby with me. I remember when Pamela was born, and they didn't give her to me right away, and I complained, I said that I wanted her right away, and one of the nurses came in and told me that they didn't give the babies right away because the mothers would tend to pick up the baby too often. And I was outraged by what she said, because I mean this was my third baby, and I wasn't supposed to know when I could pick her up, and when not to pick her up, so I spoke to the doctor, and he got kind of impatient with me for challenging the rules, and he said it had something to do with preventing infection. And I said I had been told that it was because I might not know when to pick up the baby. I guess he realized then that that wasn't very logical, so he had the supervisor come and talk to me, and I had a nice long talk with her about this whole subject of rooming-in and bonding.

When your children were sick, did you ever ask other women, or did you immediately call a doctor?

Because I had nurse friends I would sometimes consult with them. I know I would often consult with Marilyn, because she and I became very close especially around that whole issue of breast-feeding and nurturing. Marilyn was working in the same hospital as I was, and we met one day when we were walking to the hospital together. She had been watching me in the maternity outfit that I had made, and she was expecting a baby herself, and she asked me if she could borrow my uniform, because I was going to have the baby just when she was going to need one. So our whole relationship developed around our children. We had a very open relationship around how we felt about caring for our children and nursing them.

Was your church a support to your role as a mother?
I think, to be very honest, my move away from the church was precipitated by becoming a mother and what I was learning about myself and about nature. I think the church was not in touch with the natural relationship between a mother and child. I think it was because I became so much more in tune with my own self, with my nature, with the children's needs, that I found a discrepancy between that and the basic philosophy or the way people thought in the church. I certainly didn't get my support for breast-feeding from people in the church, in fact I found the opposite, there was a real resistance to it there. Becoming a mother and nurturing children was a very powerful force in my life, and I felt very much that it brought me in touch with my true nature rather than what was expected of me. I wouldn't say that's the only reason why I started to move away from the church. There's a lot of lip service given to the importance of children and how you care for them, but I didn't find that that was lived out in reality, and I really felt the discrepancy. Of course going through a divorce also strengthened that feeling.

Is it the denial of the body that the church has sometimes preached that you saw as a contradiction?
Yes. Denial of the material maybe, at the expense of the spiritual. When you deny the material, the spiritual also becomes questionable. Now you will occasionally see someone breast-feeding in church. When I was having my babies that would have been considered — well, you still hear people saying that's not natural, that shouldn't be happening.

Is there too much division made between emotional, spiritual, and physical? Were they integrated in your birth processes?
I think they were much more integrated in my own experience through the birth process and the nurturing process. The birth process is only one part of it. I wouldn't want to single out the church here, because I think most of our institutions have this problem of not integrating the whole person. The church may do it through religious dogma, but the medical profession does it through the conception of pathology and singling out a certain part of

the person, rather than looking at the whole person. And I wouldn't want to be down on the church too much, because I think there were some very positive aspects, the whole community; but if you couldn't express yourself honestly within that community, then it was very difficult to be a part of it. And certainly my children later on had a strong sense of belonging, which I couldn't share with them after a while.

How do you feel you were changed by the experience of becoming a mother?
Vastly. I think that becoming a parent is very valuable in that it helps us to work through some of our own issues. To what extent I did that at a conscious level I don't know, but I know that I experienced profound changes within myself and grew as a woman and as a person. It caused me some grief, because I didn't experience the same kind of growth in my marriage, and had a lot to do with why it didn't survive, but certainly for my own sense of myself, it was a wonderful experience.

You were a very conscious parent, I think.
Yes, I think I sort of woke up when I started to have children. I had gone through nurses' training, I'd gone through the ritual, the motions, but I never really connected with it in a very strong way, and I remember when I was at home with the children, I often thought I could never ever go back to work in an institution, because it would be too restricting. But I guess because I've had to, I have been able to some degree to integrate the kind of growth that I experienced in that period. But I think for me it was definitely a period of awakening and growth.

Would you know better now to do something differently with your children?
Oh yes, many many things I'd do differently. But I'd be much more sure of myself, much more, I wouldn't be intimidated by any kinds of social restrictions, I would go much more by my instincts and my intuitions. I remember one time my friend Marilyn calling me when she was having difficulty with her second baby, and she had this sheet in front of her that she'd been given by the hospital about nursing the baby every four hours, and I told her, "The first thing you do is throw that sheet away, and then you follow your own instincts about what you think the baby wants."

So you don't think you can imagine your life without children?
No, I can't. I mean I imagine if I hadn't had children I would have probably eventually gone on to get a Ph.D. or something like that, and my life would be different, and I would have never known what you experience when you're a mother. And whether or not the biological yearnings would have

developed, I don't know, I had my babies so early that I didn't experience that. I guess the only thing I regret, or that I wish were different for mothers, is that they would begin to value motherhood, give it some status, and that mothers who choose to be mothers and don't have the financial support of their husbands don't have to live in poverty and raise their children that way. When you look at the reality of the way most people live, many women now are sole-support parents, and they're living close to the poverty line. And that I think says a lot about our society and how we value motherhood and children and human life in general.

Aganetha (Aggie) Klassen

Aganetha (Aggie) (Ens) Klassen was born in Arkadak, Russia, in 1918. She and her husband, Menno, have five children. Aggie completed a three-year course in midwifery in Russia in two years. She lived in Neu Schönwiese, Ukraine, from 1921 to 1929, then in Einlage until her family was sent into exile in 1930 to Ural, Siberia, during the Stalinist regime. After her escape from exile in 1933 she went to Dnepropetrovsk to live with an aunt, where she remained until 1943, at which time she went to Germany. In 1947 she was able to immigrate to Paraguay. There she met and married her husband, Menno, a Canadian, and in 1949 they came to Canada. She has worked in a variety of occupations.

I have known Aggie casually for many years, but I did not know her story. As a child I heard that dreadful things happened to some of the Mennonites who remained in Russia during and after the revolution, but I cannot remember hearing anyone actually tell his or her own story in a public forum. The belief was that these things were best forgotten. Aggie does not often tell the story of her escape with her sister from Siberia, where they had been sent to do hard physical labour. The pain of mother-daughter separation in the scene where Aggie and her sister visit their mother's grave is evident in her syntax.

Aggie's personal courage and strength make her an unsung heroine. She also contributed information about her training as a midwife in Russia. Just before I left her living room, her husband came in, and the question he asked lingered with me: "Do you really think these birth stories are important?"

Do you want to start with your childhood and then talk about how you chose your profession?

OK, my childhood, what I remember, was in Neu Schönwiese [Ukraine], where I grew up. I was eleven years of age when we moved from there. Everything was taken away from my parents, because my father was a preacher and he didn't want to join the *kolkhoz* (collective farm), and so the government slowly but steadily taxed him until he had nothing left. They took our home, the house and everything else. So to save his life he disappeared to Einlage, and my sister and I stayed in the house till they had an auction sale, whatever was in the house they auctioned off, and after that we left for Einlage, where my parents were already. My father found a job as a worker, but it didn't take long, he was arrested, and for a number of months the people tried to give him a chance to get free, with the condition that he would promise never to preach. But he didn't. He loved his Lord, and he didn't intend to deny his Lord. So they said, OK, then we'll send you to Siberia. At that time there were many people that were arrested. We were put into a train and were sent into exile. In a short time my mother had to get ready. At the beginning we had some flour along and a little bit of oil, so the first year I guess was OK, but later in the year, in spring especially, we just had to go into the woods, and we had grass which we gathered, and we made soup, with no oil, no vegetables, nothing. The little bit of ration that we got I don't remember, except bread, we had 200 grams of bread. The workers got a little bit more, but it wasn't enough food for gaining strength — it wasn't enough for living and not enough for dying.

My father died of a heart attack in exile after two years, and my mother died from hunger. My oldest sister, who worked in a private home, which had other single people in exile, didn't suffer as far as hunger. So she had more energy left. And after my mother died, my sister decided we would try to escape. My older brother escaped before already which I didn't know at that time. And so my sister sold whatever we had to get as much money as we could for the trip, that was about hundred rubles. And just the day before we wanted to leave, my cousin sent us twenty-five rubles. We had a loaf of bread and a few pounds of dried fish. That was our food. But before we left, early the day before, we went to my mother's grave, and here we realized that the dogs had opened the grave which wasn't as deep as we have buried our people, the bones of my mother just left — and the rest were — the dogs — I mean the mother's body was gone.

So early in the morning we left before it was dawn and we walked about for almost three days.

Did you walk during the daytime too, or just at night?

We tried to walk during the day, too, but there we met the police, the patrol of the road, and there was only one road which led to the next train station. They took the money that we had in our little purse; the food they left, but the money they took, but the hundred rubles we had sewn in our clothes seams, so we kept them. And then they asked us to follow them, they were on a horse and buggy, and after they took a corner, we decided we would run into the forest. They didn't follow us into the forest, they left us, and we stayed until it was dark and then we walked on the road for a while, till we got to a place where someone had tried to make a mud house and it was half done, so we stayed there for the night and the next day we walked again. By the way, I was in really poor shape, I was swollen from hunger, and I was very weak too, so it was a very slow walk, we didn't progress too much, but we made a number of miles. The next afternoon it started to rain; towards the evening we were completely wet. We managed to get to a little village where we hoped someone would accept us into their home. But we knew the rules were people weren't allowed to take people in, so we prayed about it, and the first home we approached, the people allowed us to come in, and they saw our needs, and that we were very tired. They fed us and they allowed us to sleep, and then towards the evening the man of the house came in and said if we had a few rubles, there was a truck going to Sverdlovsk, where the first train station was, and we maybe could go along. So that was our saviour, shall I say, who saved us from walking many miles.

But I should go back a little bit. Before we came to this village, we were approaching a corner, and around that corner there was a hill, and on top of the hill there was the police, the guards that were supposed to stop all the people that would go by. And we knew if they would arrest us, that meant back to our exile. So both of us were really afraid, and naturally if you are afraid you just have to go to the washroom, that's what we did, and while we were there we prayed that the Lord might protect us. And I felt like in the Old Testament, where the prophet Elijah talked to his helper, who was afraid when they tried to escape, and Elijah prayed that God might open his eyes that he could see how many angels protected them from the soldiers that tried to get them, and that's what we felt it was, my first miracle that I experienced as a non-Christian at the time.

You thought of it at that time, though?

Yes. Later on it was more clear to me. Now I'll continue on from the place where we went on by truck. They covered us, because it rained first of all, and secondly for protection from the road patrol. And when we arrived in Sverdlovsk we just saw the tail of the train that we should have gone on, so we had to wait for twenty-four hours, and we were really afraid that they would approach us. But we were protected. And another thing, we were told not to buy a third-class ticket. For a second-class ticket you didn't need any documents. The third class everybody was controlled and checked for passports. So we had enough money to take a second-class ticket, and the people in that car were really kind, they realized naturally who we were; my sister was OK, but I was swollen, especially after I slept I was very swollen. And so we travelled a number of days till we got to Moscow, and in Moscow we had Mother's golden ring which we sold. We got a little bit of food, and the rest of the money we were using for our train tickets.

Did anybody approach you while you were on the train?
Not with the second class train. But in Moscow we bought again half a ticket. I was then already fourteen, but the rules were till twelve years of age you could travel by train with half a ticket. And with fourteen I should have actually had a full ticket, which we didn't have the money for, so we bought half a ticket, and I guess I looked older, but I hadn't grown since we came into exile. So we got our tickets and went to the train and went into the car in third class, and here they approached us and asked us for our train ticket as well. They didn't ask for our passports, though. And they saw me and they said, "You are older than twelve," and they threw us out of the train. So I said to my sister, "Let's try another car." We passed a few cars and went in again, and there my sister approached a person, she hoped he would help, and he did help. He said, "Have you a few rubles, maybe we can give them to the conductor that will check you," and so that's what we did, and he allowed us to stay till we had to take another train, and there we went to a market place where I had to take some clothes off and we sold them, and we added that to our train ticket, and so we got finally to our destination.

What was your destination?
At that time it was Arkadak [Saratov], where my sister knew people. She felt that because they were farmers, it would be better to stay there for a while and I would regain a little bit more strength. And then from there we left for Dnepropetrovsk, to my aunt's place, and there I stayed.

Were you in danger again, if you had been found out that you had come back?
Yes, we never told the people from where we came, where we had been, and when I came to my aunt's place, I stayed a number of months at home till she enrolled me in school, because I wasn't capable of thinking, I guess I wasn't strong enough. And there the danger was they could find out who my parents were and they wouldn't give me a passport, and I had

to receive a passport when I was sixteen. So then they asked me where my parents were, and I said they died, and that was sufficient for that time.

So this took place in 1930-33. Your life began in very troubled times, and continued that way for quite some time.
Right. Actually I never had a normal life; my childhood wasn't normal, like we call it here, let's put it that way. I never dream about those experiences, but I find it very hard to talk about the details, especially of the exile. I didn't go into the details, about how we lived, the sanitary part, it was very, very gruesome.

It must have taken tremendous courage to decide to leave, though.
I thank my sister for that. She was four and a half years older than I. She was nineteen at that time. She had the courage; but we had no choice, we knew if we would stay there, we wouldn't survive, not I. I would only have lived a month or two, not longer.

You lived for some time with your aunt in Dnepropetrovsk. What profession did you eventually study for?
My aunt helped me to choose. I always liked to help people, so there was one way of helping women, and that's why I chose to be a midwife. To help my aunt too, it was a burden for my aunt to support me, because her husband worked, she didn't, I had to be sufficient on my own. In the meantime my uncle died, while I was still studying, so I was her only relative. After I graduated from midwifery, we were asked to go into the country and work there in the smaller hospitals, where we would get our practice, not only practice, but work. To be able to graduate I had to accept 125 babies in delivery. Someone else was beside me, but I was delivering the babies. And because of my aunt being by herself, I chose to stay in the city, and I worked in a maternity hospital with newborn babies. I treated them and worked with the doctors.

Did you feel your experience there helped you when you had your own children?
Oh yes, I knew how to treat them, what to do, naturally, what you go through as a woman, so many don't know anything about their own body, which for me it was normal, ja? We studied different sicknesses of children, what was involved with children, so that was all part of it.

Did a midwife ever use anesthesia?
No. Except if you had Caesarean. No, we didn't give anesthesia if it was a normal birth.

Did they walk around while they were in labour, or were they put on a bed right away?
They walked around till they realized that was necessary.

What about forceps, were they used often?
Yes, if the woman was too narrow, then they had to be helped along, or if she was too narrow to bear the child the normal way, she had an operation.

What about episiotomies?
Yes. You see, a midwife was judged by her good performance by having the woman bear the child without tearing. It had to go a slow way, and so very few women had the problem of tearing, or they didn't cut. Except on very special occasions, and I was really surprised that that was allowed here, the fastest way. There it wasn't done the fastest way but the safest way, for the woman, for the later years, that could affect her later.

I'm interested that the midwife was judged according to how little damage the woman suffers. What else was different from your experiences?
Women were very much encouraged to nurse. There were very few ladies that didn't nurse their children. My first child was born without any anesthetic, and I could nurse her till seven months, and the rest of the children I couldn't nurse. When I worked with my hands, that affected my body, so I didn't have milk. But I always felt the anesthetic affected me. That's why I asked my doctor, and he didn't encourage to nurse, here in Canada.

How did he discourage it, or how did he put it?
Well if you can't have milk, that's OK, that's fine. He didn't try to reassure, or to make you relax, or to help along, the main thing was the child, that the child was healthy, and was fed.

There are many things that influence you, too, about nursing: if you are tense, or you have a lot of work to do.
Yes, the work, that I knew from my first child. I was washing the diapers, I had milk, but the washing, I don't know, the movement or the soap or the hot water, or whatever it was affected me. When I stopped washing diapers, my milk came back. And it was very important for us, because Karen was three weeks old when we started on our trip [from Paraguay to Canada].

Do you feel now that nursing is better, do you regret that?
I find it very important that the mother nurses the child. First of all she

gives with the milk the immunity against sickness, the children are protected more than if the mother doesn't nurse. That's all built in, and I find that's very important. But that was a new era, and I find now they encourage women to nurse, before they didn't.

Peggy Regehr

Peggy (Unruh) Regehr was born in Winkler, Manitoba, in 1928. She and her husband, Walter, have three children.

Peggy's parents were missionaries in India for many years, and Peggy spent the period from 1936 to 1942 there. She came back to North America during the war, attending schools here, and graduating with a B.A. from Tabor College (Hillsboro, Kansas). At the time I interviewed her, Peggy was Director of Women's Concerns, Mennonite Central Committee (MCC) Canada.

I first got to know her when I saw her appeal in the Mennonite Women's Concerns *newsletter for women to write about experiences in the Mennonite church or community that were unique to them. I asked her to suggest women to interview and only later realized she might have her own story to tell. My image of our interview is that of a bubbling fountain. Her voice became deeper and more confident when she told her story of employment with MCC. Peggy's narrative is confirmation that women whose needs for an outside career are not addressed during their childbearing years can and do have another chance to seize life and can refuse to be silent in response to injustice.*

When you hear the word "childbirth," what comes to your mind, and what do you feel you want to talk about first?
I guess what comes to mind first of all is my own lack of knowledge and information about anything to do with childbirth. The years that we were

in India, my mother became pregnant with the youngest in our family, my only brother, and she never shared any information about that with me. At that time I was eleven years old, I did not know that she was pregnant, I didn't notice anything different in her. I must have been terribly unobservant. And one day my mother disappeared during the night and the next day my father called us together and told us that we had a young brother. My mother never talked about childbirth or anything about the sexual aspects of becoming pregnant, so that when I went into marriage myself, I had very little knowledge of what was involved, and when I became pregnant for the first time, I guess I knew enough to know that I thought I was pregnant, but I didn't have anyone around to confirm that with me. I had done a little bit of reading here and there, although books were not easily available in those years, so I had sneaked some books, didn't let anyone know that I was that uninformed. My mother never even talked to me, really, about menstruation, for instance. I remember once she — because we were in boarding school, and I was of the age where I would probably start menstruating — she had a very short meeting with me, in which she just gave me the napkins — at that time we didn't have tampons and Kotex and all the other kinds of things that came later, we had washable napkins, and she just told me that this would probably happen, never explained to me why or the reason for it. She told me at that point never to let a man touch my breasts, and that's all the sexual information I ever received from my mother. So I was moving into something with marriage that was very strange for me.

My daughter was born ten and a half months after we were married, and I had not even gotten used to marriage before I was suddenly not feeling well. So that was a kind of traumatic experience for me. We were isolated, living out in the country in a small teacherage, a one-room country school, away from my husband's family as well as my family. I was the oldest in the family, so I was the first one having this experience. And I guess it was rather scary for me.

Pregnancy wasn't the greatest experience. I was sick the first months with all of them. And because of the kind of taboo about talking about things like that, I found that it was an uncomfortable experience, because I really was very uninformed. So especially my first pregnancy was difficult for me. We were living in a little two-room house on the same yard as another family right next to the school building, and the woman of the house had five, six children, and I guess she had noticed that I was not feeling well, and she asked me whether I was pregnant. That was right at the very beginning, and first of all I didn't want to admit it, secondly I didn't really know whether I was or not. So I said oh no no, and, I mean, she knew, [laughs] she had experienced enough of that. She was a very fine woman. I lost an opportunity of saying, "Yes, I think I am, can you tell me more?" But I was always a very fearful child through all of my life. I didn't easily talk to people I didn't know well, I didn't ask people questions. I had spent too much time in boarding school and away from my parents in isolation and without caring people around whom I could confide in, so I never learned to confide in other people. And so I really carried that by myself and struggled through it. I knew enough that I needed to go to a doctor somewhere along the line, and of course I had the regular check-ups and things like that.

Childbirth wasn't exactly celebrated either, in church circles, or in our community, was it?
Yes, it was hidden, and it was something that was expected of you. I remember at that time if you were married a year and you were not visibly pregnant, questions began to be asked of you, how come you're not having a family, what's the matter, can't you have a child, that kind of thing. As women we were expected to marry and immediately produce children because that was a woman's role. For the women in the community, it was an important event, but for the whole community it was never celebrated. You went through it yourself. If you had an extended family, then you possibly had that kind of support.

Did you let your mother know when you were pregnant, was she in India at the time?
She was in India, yes, and we let her know as soon as possible. I really can't remember her reaction. All of our communication was by correspondence, because one didn't phone across the ocean at that time. I suspect that in spite of my mother's inability to talk about sexuality, there may have been some joy, but I'm wondering whether there wasn't also some trepidation there. It's strange; there's a lot of things in my life that I don't remember. I think some of that I've blocked out because of the difficulty of my life. I don't remember anything from the first eight years of my childhood, really, until I went to India. I remember certain things about my experiences in India, probably more about the difficult experiences than the good ones. Those years in India had a tremendous impact on me.

How did you feel when you were pregnant?
I never really enjoyed the pregnancy very much. I didn't have a lot of physical problems, other than feeling nauseated. My children were all overdue, and I found the uncomfortableness and the waiting very difficult. I guess I

accepted it as part of my life, it was woman's lot. With the last pregnancy, I had a severe fall on the ice at seven months, and I had pelvic separation with that, and I ended up for the next two months being absolutely flat in bed with two small children home, and I found that very difficult; I couldn't get up for anything. The birth was very difficult, because I had been flat in bed, so all my muscles were very lax, there was no strength in them; he was also a very big baby. All my babies were big, but the last one was the biggest, he was ten pounds four ounces, and he was very long, and so it was a fairly difficult labour.

Childbirth itself was difficult in all cases. I had very long labours. And at that time, of course, women were alone, their husbands were not allowed to be there with them. I didn't have my mother around, Walter was teaching out in the country, and I was having my baby in Winnipeg, so I was taken to the hospital and left there by myself. He was not even there after the baby was born, because he was back in McTavish. And they partially drugged you at that time, so you felt out of it. I didn't feel that it was a great experience. I wasn't part of it. The first one was a very long one, and I felt very alone. I didn't know what to expect, and the nurses came in to do these things to you, they didn't explain what they were doing to you, they shaved you, they gave you enemas and did all of that kind of thing to you, and then you were left by yourself, and then you had pains, and then every once in a while they would come in to check how dilated you were, but I didn't know what they meant by "dilated," and nobody explained anything, and then finally when they thought you were ready, they wheeled you into the delivery room and they strapped you in, and gave you something, a mild amount of ether to keep you out of it. You were giving birth, but you weren't involved. And nobody sort of created an atmosphere, not even during the time that you were going for your regular appointments to the doctor, that this was something exciting to look forward to, and — I don't know. It was not — I don't know how to describe it, I'm having a very hard time thinking back, knowing how to describe it. Especially for the first one, I was very uninvolved, and a feeling like you were all alone, and nobody really cared about you as a person, it was all very medical and very mechanical around you. That doesn't mean that there weren't some fine nurses there, there were some.

They treated you as if it was an illness.

As if it was an illness, not a natural process. Nowhere had I been given any information, any sense of childbirth being a natural process. We were kept flat in bed for the first number of days, your babies were kept separate from you, they were brought in for feeding and immediately taken away again. It was something outside of us. And there's a sense in which I bonded with my children, but it wasn't easy to do that.

You could even have been brought the wrong baby, and you might not know. I would never have known. Because as soon as I gave birth the baby was wrapped up and taken out of the delivery room, I didn't even see her in the delivery room. Now with the last baby, they showed me Gerald after he was born, but with the first one, I never saw the baby until the next day sometime. And so who knows what happened.

What about breast-feeding, did you want to do it, or was it not on your agenda at all?
I wanted very much to breast-feed my daughter. I don't know where I got that from. It was going out of style at that time, but I wanted very desperately to do that. But I had not been given any kind of instruction ahead of time about how to prepare myself for breast-feeding. When my daughter was brought to me, and I tried breast-feeding her, I experienced a great deal of pain in my nipples, and that developed into sores, and I was devastated. Then I was given 292s for the pain, and then I was told — this was already after I was out of the hospital — to use the breast pump to express the milk and to feed her and then eventually it would heal and then I would be able to go back to breast-feeding. But I could not cope personally with the pain and that whole process, I spent many nights crying, and I finally gave up, with a lot of tears.

I think part of the difficulty with that was also that my daughter was born at the end of the school year, and we were going to stay in the city for the summer, and we moved into my in-laws' home. My mother-in-law had borne seven children, and this was my first child, and I felt very insecure. I didn't know how to bathe my baby, was having problems with breast-feeding, and my mother-in-law was there always looking over my shoulder. She was a very fine, caring person, but she didn't know how to support me, and instead ended up telling me what I should do, and in my insecurity, I resented that. I think if my own mother had been around, it would have been different, because I knew her. But we'd been married less than a year, I did not have a warm — I had a nice relationship! — but not a really warm relationship with my mother-in-law, and I could not take what I perceived as supervision. I also didn't know how to ask my mother-in-law for help and advice, and I tried to carry that by myself. Which, looking back, was probably silly, but recognizing the circumstances at the time, I know why I didn't ask. I can understand that. So I was thoroughly devastated by the inability to breast-feed. When my other children were born, I did not even try. I'd had such a traumatic experience that I didn't even try.

Problems with breast-feeding are common, there are ways of overcoming it, but you need to know them.
I didn't know where to go for all of that. I really feel that was in many ways because of my own childhood of being away from home so much, being in boarding schools, and then my parents going back to India when I was just barely seventeen, and being left on my own, so that I finished my high school, went through college, teaching, marriage, childbirth, everything without parents around. My siblings were still in India until the year I was married, my other sister was still down in Tabor [Kansas], going to college, so that I was very alone. My relatives were in southern Manitoba. I had an aunt who probably could have been helpful to me if there had been closer contact. We had no car at that time, we lived in the country in a small rural school. In the city I didn't know people other than my husband's family, and because the pregnancy came so early, and I hadn't built up any kinds of networking, I felt alone. But on the other hand there was also no one there who sort of tried to help me in a way that would have been helpful.

And the number of books available at that time was unbelievably poor.
It was almost nonexistent. There was Spock's child care book, on which I absolutely lived after my daughter was born, because I didn't have anyone to ask anything, and so I read it and reread it, it was my bible, my child care bible. But there wasn't very much else, there weren't books on pregnancy, on prenatal care, on what to expect, or how to prepare for breast-feeding.

Did you have anesthesia for all your births? Did you have forceps or any other medication?
I had anesthesia for all of my births. I can't remember whether forceps were used, but I suspect they were, especially in my third birth, when I had been in bed for two months and it was a very hard birth, because he was also a big baby. With my first birth, I tore badly, internally, too, and the stitches were not very well done. I experienced a great deal of pain even afterwards, when I came home. Not only was I struggling with the whole thing of trying to nurse my baby, I also couldn't stand properly, and I couldn't sit comfortably, and it took a long time for those stitches to heal. The next two births, because all my babies were large, I was cut, so that it wasn't the random tearing of the first birth, and they did a much better job of stitching me up afterwards, so that the healing was much faster. But the anesthesia, you were given enough to deaden the pain and to keep you sort of in a

floating world where you knew that there was something happening, but you weren't really part of it, and while it did deaden the pain, and with the long labour I was very tired, I still feel that being in such a foggy state at something which is such an important part of a woman's life was an injustice to me as a woman. So that I guess what came out of the whole experience for me was precisely the fact that as women we were doing something almost unnatural, that we were being treated as people who were sick, we were kept in bed long, we couldn't get up the first couple of days, and we were seen as invalids when we came back into the home, where we needed to have our mothers or our mothers-in-law there to look after us, to help us out, and where we were expected to stay at home for a longer period of time, not to go out, to protect that baby, but also for your own health, you were supposed to have a period of recovery.

You've gone back to work and experienced some reactions to that.

Let's go back half a minute. I took upon myself the traditional role of a woman, which was to stay home, to look after her children and her husband, because that was the expected role for women in our church. Women just didn't do anything else. And I accepted that role. Even though I had been a teacher before I got married, even though I had seen my mother, as a missionary, as a very strong person, who had much to give and to offer, even though I had a degree, I somehow or other let myself be hoodwinked into the idea that a woman's only role was for her family. I lived my life that way until I was fifty years old. I had begun to question that earlier, but after my children were grown, I began to think of getting out of the house and doing something, but I had gotten myself into a rut that I found I couldn't get out of. My home had become my safe place, my secure place, and the thought of moving out into society, into the world, whether to go back to school, or to work, was for me a very fearful thing.

We had talked much earlier in our marriage, when we were having a lot of financial problems, about whether I should go back to work, and I always said no, it isn't going to be good for the family, I would have to work evenings, because we didn't have child care, and that meant we wouldn't have any family life. I realize now I did a lot of rationalization already at that time. But here I had grown children who were in high school, my daughter was married, and I was still afraid of moving out of the home. And my children started putting a lot of pressure on me, and telling me that I needed to do something with my life, that I should not just stay at home. They encouraged me to find a job; well I said, what kind of a job can I have? So they said, well then at least go to school. And I rationalized that away too, I said, well my major was in business and economics, that is all outdated, the field has changed, I don't really feel like I want to go back into that field, which means I've got to start from scratch.

But they kept after me, until finally I decided that I would go back to our Mennonite Brethren Bible College part-time. I was also very afraid as an older woman, of not being able to keep up with studies at fifty years of age. I finally decided one year that I would in fact go to school, but I procrastinated until it was too late to register. But I began to realize that year what was happening to me, and the next year I did go and register.

For me that was the best thing that had ever happened in my life. Because I began to deal with issues around women's lives, and with my own life, and what had happened to me. As a member of a church that had always been very sure of what women's role was supposed to be, and that it was supported by the Bible, I began to get the theological tools for dealing with those issues, so that I could say: no, that is not all that we as women were meant to be. I also gained a lot in self-confidence as I began to recognize that I could study, that I could keep up, that I could interact with young people as an older woman and have a lot of good discussions and make good friends among the young people, and that I was accepted for who I was, not for my role as a wife and mother, but as an individual, who had something to contribute to other people.

What came out of that for me were two things: a real commitment to want to work at some women's issues, as well as a realization that I needed to do something and to move out of the home. It took several years for the right thing to come to me, but in 1984, three years after I left college, MCC (Canada) opened up a position for a half-time staff person for women's concerns. And I realized that with all of my life's experiences, and with all I had learned theologically, and with some of the gifts and abilities I had, that that was the right position for me, and so I applied for that position. It was only a half-time voluntary service position when I started, which meant that I was paid a small allowance, but I was not paid a salary. I was willing to do that for a two-year term, but for me coming out of that was also the issue of how we have expected women always to be the volunteers and the men were the ones who got paid.

When I got that position, I went to my church and spoke to my pastor about my job, and asked for an opportunity to share with the church something about it, so that I could also experience the support of my congregation. Within the church we allow people who go into various kinds of church ministries to share on a Sunday morning where they are going, and then as a church we give our blessing to those people, we let them know that they will have our support. And he was very hesitant about doing it, feeling that women's issues were much too touchy, not being sure that that was the right kind of thing to do, sharing his own discomfort with my position, and saying, maybe somewhere along the line he would do that, but he would see first, he would talk to some other people. I never got the opportunity to do that, and I never had the support of my church for my work, even though it's church-related work, and I was dealing with issues about women, who make up over half of the membership of our churches. Even today, many people in my church congregation do not know that I am working in this position, and are surprised when after four and a half years they find that I have been working for that long with MCC, which is a well-respected organization within our churches. If we had sent an MCC volunteer overseas, we would have made a big thing about it, but because I was dealing with the kind of program that I was doing, and because I was moving into a position of leadership within a church structure, it was in a sense new for at least my own Mennonite conference. Of course, women from the church have worked for a long time, and we have many women in our church who have gone back to work. Not young women with small children, mostly older women whose children are already grown up, and that has been an accepted phenomenon. But I think it was the fact that I was dealing with the kind of issues that I was dealing with, and that I was in leadership position within a church organization, which was the stumbling block for expressing interest in what I was doing and support for me in my program.

We are slowly moving towards having more women in program areas, but we still do not want to tackle the issues that come with women in an organization being ghettoized mostly at the lower level, at the secretarial and clerical level. Most of the people in the administrative and program areas of the organization are salaried men, and often most of the people who are on voluntary service within the organization are women at the lower level. And the salary scales. There is such a wide range between the women who are doing most of the lower-level jobs and the men who are doing the higher-level jobs. As I've tried to address some of those issues I have found that I'm treading on toes and have experienced resistance to what I am doing, unwillingness to tackle those issues, and in fact have taken some personal attacks and personal criticisms about what I am doing.

We are very strong on justice issues for other people, and we don't know how to deal with justice issues within the organization. We are very strong on models of mediation and conciliation out in society, but we have been resistant, as I have asked for, occasionally, to accept mediation and conciliation for resolving differences within the organization. For me that has been very disillusioning, for an organization that I deeply respect and have put so much of my time and energy into. It is also a problem for me to move from voluntary service to salary. Most men, when they start on voluntary service, after two years they say that they need their expertise to continue and then are put on salary. After two years, I asked for salary, I was rejected. A year later I again asked for salary, and was rejected. But at that time I did not allow the issue to die. I made it a justice issue, feeling that I needed to be treated the same way that men were treated. I was told that I did not need a salary because I had a husband who supported me. And so eventually, my supervisor and I decided that — no, he decided that the only way that he would deal with that issue, since he and I could not resolve it, would be to go to arbitration. I wanted mediation rather, feeling that maybe we could come to a compromise situation. But he did not want that, he wanted both of us to state our cases to a forum of three people who would then decide between our respective positions, and I think that he thought that he had the stronger position. The decision went for me, in terms of giving me salary. Even there, I found myself willing to compromise, I was willing to put that off for another six months. So that I had worked almost four years before I finally got salary. Shortly after that, the process began that eventually pushed me out of the organization. So that I feel that my pushing for justice and for salary for myself also created a backlash, and the process began in which eventually I found myself being given a limited term instead of a three-year term in order to terminate me. Which would make it look not as if I had been fired, but which in essence was a firing.

And you have no recourse to anybody?
I have tried all the recourses, and I have not been able to get any justice. I have come to realize that organizations and institutions can be abusive, just as we can have abuse in the home. It's an institutional abuse, it isn't abuse of one person over another, but it is a power and a control issue, and there is victimization, just as there is victimization in spouse abuse. And I have learned a lot about spouse abuse in working with that issue within the organization. And the blaming of the victim. And keeping the person always insecure by not communicating what is going on. Some day I want to write something on institutional abuse, and apply it very specifically to churches and church institutions, so that it will be helpful to us within the church. But I think I need first of all to overcome some of my own anger and frustration before I can do something that will be helpful.

Women still are kept powerless. We are not treated equally with men as people who can make adequate decisions about ourselves. And if we come across differently than in that very fine, gentle, feminine way that we were taught to be — except that many of us weren't that way, neither my mother nor my grandmother was a very gentle person, they were strong people, and I've inherited some of that from them, even though I've always been a very insecure, very afraid person — we find no acceptance of ourselves, we are then those abrasive women, who are trying to push their way into places of power, or to be like men, or who hate men, all kinds of accusations are thrown against us.

The fear is that we will use the power that we gain in the same way they have used it, over other people.
That's right. And one of the things that I am discovering is that women have a much different concept of power. It's the concept of empowerment, not of a limited amount of power that if it's diluted too much and spread among too many people, we'll all have too small amount of it, but rather the concept of empowerment, where each one of us is empowered to make decisions about our own lives, and to use who we are as people in some kind of way to be a benefit, to society, to the church, to our families. And women are coming together in many different ways, in small groups, networking, where they are empowering each other, in women's conferences, where they operate on a very different basis, where they come for some mutual support and acceptance of one another.

I'm curious: do you have an idea of where you want to go from here then?
No, I don't. At this point I don't. First of all I was devastated by this experience, and it has taken me a long time to deal with that devastation. I have a lot of ideas —

Do you feel that maybe women have to divorce themselves from institutions and begin to work from the outside to change things?
That's one of the things that I'm considering doing. There are benefits to working within the institutions, part of which is the finances that you have in order to do the kinds of things that you want to do, and the good will that there often is for the institution, so that it creates openings for you. When you're on your own, you neither have the finances nor do you have the natural inroads into the areas that you would like to penetrate. On the other hand, I think that there is much that one can do from outside. And one of the things is work, to a certain extent, with greater integrity. You no longer have to be so conscious of the fact that the organization is dependent on a constituency for its finances, and if you overstep certain bounds, and say something a little too strongly, you will affect the organization doing its many good things. So there are some definite advantages to that. For me, in

wanting to do that, the difficulty will be precisely in trying to find the finances for that. Having been in the home most of my life, having been paid salary here for eleven months, having a husband who's retired and on pension right now, there isn't a lot of extra money. And so while I have a lot of ideas, I think I need some distance first of all from my experience here, and then I need to start putting those into a hopper and find out where I can go with those. It may be working very specifically on women's issues, and finding some way of doing it on my own, or trying to move back into another institution, though I'm not sure that I could find the right place for myself.

Edith Parker

Edith (Falk) Parker was born in Herbert, Saskatchewan, in 1931. She and her former husband, Clare, had two children. When I spoke with her she was Director of Maternal Child Nursing at St. Boniface Hospital in Winnipeg.

Edith Parker was introduced to me by a nurse-midwife at the hospital, Kris Robinson, who said to me, "You could interview the director of nursing on the obstetrics floor, Edith Parker." "Oh, but I'm only interviewing Mennonite women," I replied, not thinking of the fact that Mennonite women who marry lose their names. Edith Parker was born into a Mennonite home in Saskatchewan and recalls a home birth on her parents' farm when a couple was forced by a winter storm to stay overnight at their place. From Edith I was able to get a picture of what has changed and what has not changed on the maternity floor since I was a woman in labour in 1962. It was a pleasure to interview someone who knew the labour floor from the point of view of the caretakers rather than the consumers of their services.

Edith, you talked briefly last time about a birth on a farm that you were going to tell me about.
Yes. At the time we were living north of the little town of Herbert in a farming district, and my uncle lived just a mile from us. The particular birth that I was talking about occurred in 1937, when I was a small child. It was in the dead of winter, we just had had a snowstorm and we were all

snowed in. However, my mother had planned to have guests that Sunday, my uncle and his family were coming over, but she was interrupted in her preparations for the noon meal with a man coming to our door, and he spoke to my mother in Low German. They had come from ten miles further north and were on their way to the little town of Herbert, his wife was in labour, and was about to give birth. So one of my brothers was dispensed to the barn to tell my dad that there was a problem, and my oldest brother was told to go and find a second team of horses, hitch it to one of the sleighs, and bundle all the younger children into the sleigh and go over to Uncle John's and tell him that they couldn't come over for dinner that day, and also that there was something rather dramatic going on at our house. So my dad came from the barn, and in the meantime my mother had welcomed the woman into the house. I can see her yet, as she was starting to take out clean sheets and prepare a bed in the living room, right beside the heater. My dad and the man took the bobsleigh and went to town to fetch the doctor. In the meantime, we went off to our uncle's, and my mother was left with my oldest sister, she was about fifteen, sixteen at the time, and my brother who was about three or so. To this day I don't know how my mother had the good sense to do it, but she got some string sterilized and a pair of scissors and some boiling water, and then she proceeded to deliver this baby, who was coming, whether we wanted him or not! I mean, the woman delivered the baby, my mother simply assisted her, and supported her, so that she wouldn't get too panicky. I think my mother probably was more frightened than the patient was at that time. It was a healthy baby boy, my mother cut the cord, and made sure the placenta was delivered, and had the good sense to save it for the doctor to examine. So the doctor came, and he checked the woman, who had been comfortably settled in the bedroom by that time. The little cradle that had been used for the last child a few years ago was brought out, and the baby put in it beside the mother in bed, and the doctor gave his approval, and said there wasn't any point in moving the patient. My mother and father agreed, in spite of the fact we had a rather small house with a big family. The lady was then put into this bedroom with her child, and we had to move out into the living room, and sleep on the floor for the week she was there! The patient did very well, and the family was so delighted that the child's second name was after my father, Jacob William.

Do you attribute your choice of profession to this incident?
Another baby was always welcome. I had the distinct feeling with this child that was born so precipitously at our house, that my mother never questioned, and neither did any of us, that this woman and her child

shouldn't be looked after; we just assumed that this baby was very precious, and we were all excited when we came back from Uncle John's, and we were given the privilege of looking at this new baby. So my feeling towards birth and that was always positive.

Did your mother tell you about births in her generation at all?
Very little, although I think my mother probably told me more than many Mennonite mothers did. The farm is a great education for youngsters, because even though the young children were often shooed away, we were still there for the birth of a calf, or the birth of piglets, and I think that it was never a feeling of great apprehension, that this was something that should be put out of the context of normal, everyday living.

Then shall we jump to the birth of your children?
I had done my nurses' training at the Grace Hospital. They had, for the size of the hospital, a very large obstetrical department, and I had thoroughly enjoyed obstetrics. I went back to have my first child at the same hospital, and at that time, things were pretty rigid. Husbands weren't in delivery rooms, and were discouraged even to stay with you in labour. My first labour was very long, and probably, if I had not had a friend with me, I would have got very discouraged. Bonnie was not an obstetrics nurse. And that's why I think it's so important, that another woman be with a labouring woman. She came in, she looked at my husband who was sitting there, and said, "You look terrible. Why don't you go home and have a cup of coffee, and when you feel better, you can come back." And the look of relief that went over his face, when Bonnie took hold, and I started relaxing. I really started progressing in labour once Bonnie was with me. And she did say, "I think you could have an analgesic now. Maybe that would help you a little further." It was an analgesic that was quite appropriately given, so it worked very nicely without making me drowsy or unable to know what was going on. And then she said, "Do you feel like pushing yet?" and I said, "No, not really, but maybe I'll try with this contraction," and I wasn't really that uncomfortable. And she said, "Oh, I think I'll go for the nurse, I think I'm beginning to see the top of his head." The baby had been in what we call a posterior position, and all of a sudden, with her being with me, I was able to get that baby turned around. And lo and behold, by the time she'd got the nurse, and they had me transferred onto a stretcher and taken me to the case room, the anesthetist came in, and I said, "Oh, I don't want anything." And he said, "Well, you better stop pushing, because you're going to have this baby before the doctor gets here!" [laughs] Fortunately my doctor was only about five or ten minutes from the hospital. In the end, after about

twenty-four hours of labour, this was a relatively easy birth, after the baby turned, and what was so marvellous is that I was fully awake. It was a great experience, a very exhilarating experience. I felt involved, more so than I did with my second child.

For the second baby, I actually had some anesthetic, which I didn't really want, but again, she was posterior, and she didn't turn on her own. And that probably was due to the fact that the analgesic wasn't administered at the right time, and I was too drowsy to do the pushing afterwards. It was two o'clock in the morning, and so the forceps were applied, and when I woke up, they said, "You have a beautiful daughter." And it's interesting how patients respond. I didn't think of this beautiful daughter, I said to the doctor, "*You* put me out!" It was strange, it was almost a reflex response: I remember seeing my son, and being wide awake, and you didn't give me that chance with my daughter. I've thought of that often, when we do this to patients. It doesn't happen too often any more, but it used to happen, without discussing it with them, and saying, look, I'm going to have to use forceps. Now of course we have epidurals, usually, so that at least patients are very much involved, even when forceps have to be applied.

What about breast-feeding?
Fortunately I had a physician who said there was no other way. [laughs] We in North America have always been far less pro-breast-feeding than the European and also the United Kingdom, and this particular physician took his post-graduate training in Ireland, so there was no other way! And he was so thoroughly convinced that breast-feeding was right, he would not ever prescribe any sort of drug to dry it up. I think that, too, is very important. Sure, I think there's the odd woman who for one reason or another doesn't successfully breast-feed a baby, at least for a six-week period, or longer than that, but most of it has to do with attitudes of care givers, and attitudes of the patient herself, and also having the understanding that this is something you work at, it doesn't arrive immediately. There's all sorts of flexibility involved, it's not a system that says in three hours this child has to eat, or in four hours this child has to eat, and the more you feed, the more the milk production is stimulated. A lot of these things we didn't know, so there wasn't that help available. So I think I probably would not have breast-fed if I hadn't had such a determined physician. I just automatically fell into place with his wishes. But that was the thing, a lot of women had physicians who did not advocate it, and automatically we did as the physician said.

I know you're talking personally, but what changes have you seen in the labour wards?
Just as a qualifier, many of the opinions that I will present to you here, I

speak as an individual who has been involved in the maternal child and obstetric care for a long period of time. Sure, some of my experiences come as a Director of Maternal and Child Nursing, but they're really more personal. I'd like to go back a little further, because I worked as the obstetrical supervisor at the Grace Hospital from 1966 on, and I have seen many changes since then. I recall the first time a physician — I don't think he'd mind if I mentioned his name, it was Dr. Blouw — came to me, and he had this patient who wanted her husband present for a delivery. People just didn't do that in most hospitals at that time. This was 1967 or '68. So I got this letter from the administrator of the hospital saying that Dr. Blouw had requested this. And she said, "You're not going to do that, are you?" And I said, "Well, I don't really see what's wrong with it. If the doctor doesn't mind, nurses certainly don't mind. And husbands can sometimes be a very big support to their wives." So we had the husband in for delivery. I remember going to a meeting with some of my peers one time, and I was introduced and they said, "Oh, you are the woman who let husbands into the delivery room, aren't you!" At the time I felt almost as if I was being attacked about it by other care givers, but since then we have all accepted that as normal, and we encourage husbands to feel comfortable with that notion. We also had some dire predictions of husbands fainting and falling. One nurse said, "Oh, he's going to faint for sure!" and I said, "Where are you putting him?" "Well, he wants to see everything!" and she was complaining about this, so I said, "No, no, no. What is the objective of the husband being there? He wants to be there because he wants to share this experience with his wife, he wants to support her during a time when he feels she's under a great deal of stress. And so we position him so he can support her. That is, putting him right beside her head, where she's hearing what he's saying, and we don't tie her hands down, we let him hold her hand instead, and we make him comfortable and sit him on a stool, and if he should feel faint, he can just put his head down briefly." When I go to the labour floor here now, I see a nurse saying, "I'll show you where you change now, we're just about ready for this delivery." And in the birthing room, husbands become very much part of the delivery. In the birthing room they don't move at all, they just stay in that one room. And certainly I think anybody planning new facilities would plan on that kind of a set-up, because actually it's cost-effective, too. I really believe that things like mother/baby/couple care, birthing rooms don't have to be elaborate, it has more to do with attitude of the care givers than it does with the physical plant. I don't think you need queen-size beds and beautiful draperies — it's nice if you have them, but if the right attitude exists with the care givers, whether it be nursing staff, house physician, house staff, or the physicians themselves, then this can be a good experience. I think why St. Boniface may be important to couples, too, is that while they want this very original experience for themselves, they also want to make sure that all the safety nets are in place. And where you have a neonatologist, where you have an anesthetist, you know that those factors will be looked after as well. The care givers have a responsibility, if the couple has to face, for instance, switching from a normal delivery to the woman having a Caesarean delivery.

You've mentioned that couples will shop around, and you think there are some reasons why they choose St. Boniface sometimes.

I think couples are much better informed than they used to be. It's no longer "the woman is having a baby." This family is having a baby. Couples do a lot of planning for having their children — you see this particularly in the professional group, in the middle class, upper middle class area — they have a definite goal in mind, and they wait probably till a little later to have their family, then they want to have these two perfect kids. And they want this to be a meaningful experience. So they shop around and consider, do they have things like a neonatologist available, if something should go wrong, do they have an anesthetist, if I need an epidural for some reason or other, could I have that kind of therapy as well; also, how rigid are they? And they come in with their birth plans, and they may have a list of things that they want done, and that's great. Sometimes I'll have couples that phone me directly and I will say, "Now look, when you have your birth plan, you send it in, we'll put it into your file, and we have a prenatal sheet on you which your doctor probably will submit to us, and when you come in, you just tell the admitting nurse that you have submitted your birth plan, so she will look for it then. And if you happen to get a nurse that's sort of discouraging, then just say, 'But I was told all this was available,' and that's all." When we were moving into this whole notion of couples participating in the decision-making with regard to the birth, it took a lot of reinforcement. We also saw the gradual changing in the staff. As the younger nurses came, of course, they didn't know anything else, and it was much easier for them to fit in. The more nurses we got who had this kind of thinking that this is a couple's great experience, they want to make it worthwhile, so we want to allow them to do it in their own way; we have found that it's easier to allow couples to do this.

We talked earlier about the changes that have taken place on the labour floor, for instance that women don't have to lie down, they can walk around, and so on. What other changes have there been on the labour floor?

We used to give patients enemas, we used to do shave preps, and now many times we don't do any of the shaving prep any more, we might do what we call a very mini prep, and if any enemas are given, it might be the woman's choice to have a small Fleet enema, just to help her, if she feels that she has needed that. But there's much more choice, and there isn't this sort of rigid protocol: This is what we do. And I don't think we really thought of how uncomfortable we made women feel sometimes. We went through the stage in the early seventies, when we had the fetal monitors, they were the be-all and the end-all, we based everything on this fetal monitor. And gradually we've gone past that, we had to have another look at the fetal monitoring. It's just another tool to help us look at this baby and see how he's doing, and how he or she is tolerating the labour. And also to see how Mother's labour is, whether it's effective, and so on. For instance, if a woman has had a Caesarean delivery before, and it would not necessarily be duplicated in the second pregnancy, we would then give her a trial of labour. We find we are doing this much more frequently, and that of the women who have had previous Caesarean deliveries, and opt for a trial of labour the second time around, somewhere between sixty to seventy percent, closer to seventy percent manage to deliver vaginally. I think we progressed through the seventies, and hopefully in the latter part of the eighties we have taken this a step further and said, technology is an asset. But it does not rule, the patient and the care giver still have to make the decisions. And clinical decisions should not be based on what one machine tells you. That's being simplistic. Also, I think we've seen a positive impact on Caesarean delivery rates, that we were actually able to lower the rates we had when we were looking just at the fetal monitor. And it's true. I used to find that I would go in when the junior staff was with a patient, and yes, the sad part was that sometimes they were nursing the machine, and not the patient.

But I see the excellent nurse or the very experienced nurse-midwife, and we have quite a few British-trained midwives in our department, who assess the patient, and the patient has all sorts of choices, to get up, to move around, to be held by the nurse, to sit, to squat; we are much more open to choices.

I think nurses are more on the forefront of change than the doctors; you seem to know better what the patient, or the person who comes to you, needs.

I remember in one managing course reading an article in which the writer compared hospitals to feudal systems, where we have the peons and all the way up to the knights and so on and so forth, and the physician was the lord of the manor. And in many ways this is true. As a student I recall being required to rise when the physician came through the nursing station. This of course has changed very dramatically, and I don't feel that I'm a nurse who's called a doctor-basher, that everything's wrong with the medical profession. But for very many years, physicians were taught they were the ultimate makers of all health-care decisions, and life-and-death decisions, and to a certain extent that message is still given in the medical schools, not as much, because we're starting to see even in the selection of medical students things like maturity and empathy and these sort of attitudes being assessed, as far as the applicants are concerned, not just whether these were the "A" students, and that was it. And I think that that's a very difficult thing for a physician to give up, because it is tied up with power. For many, many years, members of the medical profession have seen themselves as the power brokers in the health care system. And that's a spot that nobody wants to give up, they had it for so long, you went into medicine because you wanted to control these things. So I'm not too surprised.

Nurses, on the other hand, have always come from the other side, usually hospital nursing schools were connected to religious organizations, and somehow we were taught that the last shall be first, and we should be very humble, and we should serve, and for that reason we're not coming from the same base, that we need to be constantly in control. We did have to change with the starched uniform and the bibs and aprons and the hard collars we used to wear as student nurses, and as we changed the uniforms, we gradually changed people. Even now I sometimes say to some of my staff, having spent some time in public health nursing, "I wish you'd all go and make a public health visit sometime. Because when you knock on that door, and the client lets you into her house, you're on her territory, and she's giving the orders, you aren't. You're asking her whether you can come into her territory."

Another thing is that nurses have been largely female. And of course this came from the notion of nurturing and caring and supporting and so on. A physician from Case Western did a large study in Guatemala on bonding between the mother and child. This was a sequence to the earlier bonding studies that he had done, but this involved a large patient sample, thousands and thousands, and they found that if a woman had somebody with her throughout her labour, the labour was significantly shorter, she seemed to bond more easily with her child, and the significant part that they found over and above somebody always being with the patient, was that another woman seemed to have the most beneficial effect. And if we look at the development of midwifery, and even of the story I told you right at the start, it was really the knowledge of the woman in the neighbourhood that got called in, and I think from there originated the notion of midwives, the midwife was helping the woman to deliver this baby.

What would you say to your own daughter?
I would say, particularly if she waited till after thirty to have her babies, yes, you have to go to a centre where everything is available, should an intervention be needed, that it is there. As a professional in the obstetrics field, I also know the physicians around that I feel would allow her the choices and still provide the standard of care that she should have, so I would of course encourage her to go to that kind of physician. But I would also tell her to demand things, like a birthing room, unless there was some really marked high-risk factor.

Is there anything else you wanted to say?
Well, just that I never get past the marvel of birth, and new life. For me it's a privilege to see all the changes, but to know that in some things we're coming right back to the basics, which were important. That babies are important, women are important, that couples together deliver this baby, and that care givers are merely there to assist them.

SUE KLASSEN

Sue (Wallace) Klassen was born in Wilmington, Delaware, in 1960 and now lives in Webster, New York. Her husband, Robert Victor, is my nephew. They have two children. Sue, an honours graduate from the University of Waterloo, is now a homemaker who runs a family day-care in her house.

In November 1988 I was in Toronto for family reasons and I stayed a few extra days to interview Sue, Magdalene Redekop, and Hildegard Martens. At the time I interviewed Sue, she had borne one child at home in Waterloo, Ontario, with the help of two midwives, Elsie Cressman and Francesca (surname unknown). In the hour we spent together, I again had the rush of energy that I had experienced before and was beginning to expect whenever I interviewed. I do not consider myself to be a mystical person — I like to pin down facts — but more and more when I sat down with women to hear their birth stories, a sense of reverence entered the interchange without any conscious effort on our part. Sue had a slight headache and would have liked to cancel, but since I had come from a distance and was counting on her she went ahead. By the time we finished, her headache was gone. Unfortunately, I accidentally erased half of Sue's tape. We later tried to redo the tape, but we agreed that it was not possible to re-create the interview.

How did you choose your doctor?
Elsie Cressman had said that I absolutely had to have a doctor, and one

supportive of home birth. I had been to a woman physician, a general practitioner, a few times. When I asked if she would be open to the possibility of supporting somebody through home birth, she said no. Elsie had the names of two physicians in town that were possibilities, and I chose one who worked a lot where the Old Order people live, but who was very far from the Old Order tradition himself. He shared office space with another young doctor, who drove a motorcycle and wore a black leather jacket, who also worked with the Old Order Mennonites, and there was a picture of a body builder on the wall of the office! [laughs] Some contradictions, but the Old Order people come in here happily. It's neat to see these meshings, and that a lot of values can be shared. We have been very happy with this doctor's use of technology. He is aware of all the medical literature, we've found his explanations very clear about what is happening, but he uses simple methods to deal with things, rather than complex ones, when it's helpful. For example, when I had a yeast infection, the midwife recommended using yogurt on a pad to fight that, and he recommended changes in diet, and the combination has been very effective.

So you saw both a midwife and a doctor.
Yes. I was far better taken care of than my hospital birth counterparts, because initially I saw Elsie every month, and Dr. A. every two months at the beginning. Towards the end I was seeing someone every week, and towards the very end I had two very competent midwives, and a competent doctor. I chose not to have an ultrasound, because there is little evidence that it gives you any positive information. It gives you a brief moment of fun, looking at the picture of your baby moving, but I thought, I can do without that brief pleasure, when we don't know about the results of ultrasounds. So I felt very positive about the pregnancy. Early on we told both sets of parents, I guess somewhere around six or seven weeks along. I have always been relatively open with my parents, and they have always encouraged us to form our own views, but they have always told us the reasons for theirs. I think Victor was a little shocked when I immediately told them that we were planning to have a home birth if the pregnancy went along well, and that we had a midwife. My parents had some very deep concerns, and Victor said afterwards, "Why did you tell them, we haven't had a chance to do all the reading, to be prepared with the refutes." My mother in particular was concerned, because her first child died at four days old from heart problems, her second child had an ovarian cyst, I was her third child, the fourth child was fine as well, and the fifth child had spina bifida, hydrocephalus, and would have died without prompt medical treatment. So she had very direct reasons to have concerns. But I had read

about these things and felt very comfortable. We live twenty minutes from a hospital, and it probably takes that long to gear up the major surgery anyway. So in time we did answer those questions for my parents. One book, *Midwifery is Catching*, is one that I lent my mother, and Michel Odent's *Birth Reborn*. She became a very positive supporter, or at least accepted that our decision could be a good one. She had never minded her hospital births, she had had positive experiences, and never minded being cut or anything, she had just accepted it all and still has no negative feelings. My father was I think a little more open to the idea from the beginning, and was quite positive about it. Victor's parents were somewhat hesitant, but certainly nobody was putting a foot in the way of us. And I never really had any problems with anybody giving us a lot of negative feedback, I suppose because I felt very confident myself, and I never made a big deal out of it. If anybody asked, I would mention that we were planning to have it at home, and there might be a little silence, but we were never militant about it, and nobody was militant in return. I guess I've always tended to be different! After the fact, people have been really curious about it, and we've talked about it a lot with a lot of people, who have been really fascinated by the whole thing. I never thought it was anything too strange, because I'd never given birth any other way. I did a lot of reading during pregnancy, and the more reading I did, the more positive I felt about the beauty of the God-given mechanism to give birth, and how it is all in such a beautiful balance, but a delicate balance, one that is very easily tipped by many things. So I am glad to keep technology out of it as long as possible, but welcome the advantages that can be given when that balance has already been tipped.

Very early in my pregnancy I had to come to terms with accepting the child that was within me, not knowing what that child would be, anything about that child, whether that child would have multiple deformities, be perfect, be a girl, be a boy, be inclined towards academics. The greatest thing was that three of my mother's five children had had birth abnormalities. I could not put off that possibility as something that happens to other people, or to bad people, or to people who don't take care of themselves. My mom was a home ec. teacher, nutrition was extremely important to her, she raised us as healthfully as she knew how, and three of her five children had moderate to severe difficulties. So I *had* to deal with that, and I *was* able to deal with that, finally, at a very deep level. It's one thing to deal with it in your head, and it's a very different matter to deal with it deep in your heart. But I am very thankful to God for that deep peace and acceptance of the child within. I wrote a lullaby in the car one day, and I still sing it to him. It was a prayer as well as a lullaby. And at a very deep level, there was acceptance. Still, occasionally I felt the waves of concern or anxiety that we all feel, but at the deepest level there was a peace. Just before Christmas, a month or two before Nathan would be born, I was asked by a girl in my church: "So you must be scared, eh?" and I thought, I used to be! I used to be so afraid, my initial feelings were ones of very deep fear. And I thought, how that has changed! I stopped and pondered that for probably several minutes, and I said, "No, I am not afraid. I have a deep peace about it. And the more I've read, the more I trust in the body's ability to give birth, and the grace of God to be there, no matter what, to be watching over. If it does not go the way I might hope, He is there, strengthening, supporting, making beauty out of what happens."

We had a wonderful summer, because I wasn't working, and I was only going to be teaching half-time. I was aiming towards being home and making that transition. So I sang a lot, we went on a canoeing trip, we went on a backpacking trip. I was starting to be uncomfortable in my regular clothes at two and a half months, and I was out of them at three and a half months, even though I had lost five pounds from my pre-pregnancy weight. I was eating all the time, huge amounts, but I wasn't gaining weight, I was getting lots of exercise, and eating lots of carbohydrates, and so on. So it was a very joyful pregnancy. I've never felt so healthy in my life, we had a wonderful time. We even did skiing in the winter, we didn't do big hills, just little grades.

You skied the morning that you gave birth, didn't you?
Well, yeah, I guess it was the Thursday night, we went out skiing for about half an hour. Victor said, "I wish we'd gone out earlier, because we could have had a long enough ski." It was a little dark by the time we got back to the car, and it just wasn't safe. At four in the morning, my water broke. This was two weeks before the, quote, due date, but it was funny, I had tried to expect him three weeks late, because I thought it's much easier to have him early than late, and I didn't want to be chafing at the bit and anxious. So I tried to gear up for three weeks late, and he actually came two weeks early. Well, in the couple of days before he was born, I had intense heartburn. I had eaten papaya to help quell heartburn occasionally, but it was beyond papaya, and there was no way I was going to take any medication. And I was praying, gosh, five more weeks of this! I don't know that I can stand it! God — you'll be with me! But this feels tough! And then suddenly the baby was on its way. When my water broke, I put in more pads, and I went and wrote in the mother's journal that Mom Klassen had given me, and then I planted a little kiss on Victor's forehead, and mentioned in a quiet little voice, "I'm in labour." I wanted him to go right back to sleep, I didn't want to disturb his sleep at four in the morning, but I just wanted to mention it,

in case he wasn't sleeping, too. Well, that kind of did it for sleep for him.

We went out for a walk at about six in the morning. I had already taken castor oil to clean out my bowels, so that I didn't have to have any enemas. It was a beautiful morning, the snow was coming down, just perfect! We went for a long walk, on our forty-five minute walk that we took every evening, and got about halfway around, and the castor oil had worked! There was no way I was going to be able to get home. We saw a man out snow shovelling, and I had to ask him, "Excuse me, I'm sorry, I'm in labour, and I really have to go to the bathroom. I wondered if I could use your toilet." He stopped, leaned on his shovel, and looked and looked for a long minute. I don't think he could put it all together! Here's this huge woman, I mean huge tummy. And he says, "OK, you can go down and use the one in the basement, but the kids are sleeping, so go quietly." So I went, and I was in there a long time. But when I came out, he said, "So when are you expecting?" And I said, "I'm in labour right now." And he looked for another *long*, long time, and he said, "Well — good luck." I think he thought we were very unusual!

We got home and phoned Elsie. She was in the middle of another birth giving, so she came out after that. I wasn't dilated highly at all, I had a *long* way to go. I had been to the midwife the afternoon before, just before we went skiing, and she said to me, "You've got a good big baby in there, there's no room left, ready to come any time." And it seems like he ran out of room and decided to come, but he was coming slowly. Around ten in the morning was the lowest time, because it didn't seem like anything was happening, and that was discouraging. But Elsie explained that this was necessary, those first ones were not the real working ones, they really had to be ten minutes apart before they could start doing the work, and then they could get more frequent. So we followed her recommendation. I took a short nap in the afternoon, and was eating when I felt like it. Around five o'clock Mom Klassen and my Oma brought over chicken noodle soup. By then I was starting to get contractions that I had to think about. I would have a spoonful and go and have a contraction, sort of lean in against the stairs, it helped to sort of kneel on the stairs, I did a lot of my labour on the stairs. But it was nice to be able to walk around and do things freely and have different places.

Labour was beautiful. It was hard, I have never worked so hard in my life. It was not comfortable. But it wasn't something I would really call pain, certainly not searing pain, not sudden pain. It took absolutely all of my concentration, it took absolutely everything within me, I was making primeval noises, deep groans, and calls, but interspersed with that were the moments when I would think, Oh, joy! I felt joy, I felt no fear when labour actually was under way. Victor rubbed my back through every contraction. He had like forty seconds to eat in between, and then he had to be back on the job. My midwife suggested that I go into the tub, that was *awful* for me, it was just the wrong thing for me, because of the way he was coming down, I guess every baby is different. Squatting on the toilet did help, and being on the stairs did help. I was still going quite slowly, and at seven at night, Elsie was going to give a slide show in some town, quite a drive away. Francesca was there, and Elsie said, "Is it OK for me to go?" And I said, "Yeah, go, we'll page you if things happen really fast."

Well that's when things started really happening! We called there just as she'd got *in*to the slide show, she hadn't given any part of it, and she had to turn right around and come back. That's the life of a midwife, it must be very hard. She came right back, and arrived about three minutes before Nathan's head came out. They had a mirror, so I could see Nathan's head coming out. I actually pushed on the bed. I had contemplated doing it standing up, but it's just not as stable, and it didn't feel comfortable to get on the bed. And this was the most intrusive part of the whole thing, they started putting hot compresses on me and stretching my perineum, and wanting me to sit down. They didn't interrupt my concentration by talking, except when I said ouch! The only time I said ouch was when they were stretching my perineum. And I thought, OK, but I want that to be done. The thing that felt really intrusive was when they told me to *wait* when I wanted to push, wait till they checked out how dilated I was. And I thought, I *cannot wait!* You know, everything within me wanted to push! But basically they sat off in the corner, they occasionally made suggestions, but they were just *there*, as a source of strength and support and guidance, but quiet and waiting. Letting the body do it. And it was just beautiful to see the head push out. But to show how much I was in a different state, pushing and pushing, I could see the top of the head coming, and finally the head comes out, the midwife helps to turn the head around, and I exclaim, "It has a face!" [laughs] Just totally in a different world.

Anyway it was just beautiful, and Nathan came out, and he was placed immediately on my tummy, and I thought, Hurry up, I want him on my breast! But then Victor cut the cord, and after it had stopped beating, it was clamped and he cut it, and then Nathan was at my breast, and he was awake for three and a half hours after he was born at nine that night, he nursed for about three hours of that time. After he had nursed for an hour, they asked if they could do a quick weigh, and they did that gently, they hung him in a blanket off a spring scale, and he was washed up a little bit while I got into the tub and washed off. But while I was in the tub I had him back on the breast, and it was just so beautiful, it was just so right. And then around eleven o'clock Victor's family came over, and he was still nursing away, hungry little guy! I allowed each of them to hold him, but not for long, because the kid wanted to nurse again! [laughs] and finally he went back to sleep. So it was beautiful.

Magdalene Redekop

Magdalene (Falk) Redekop was born in Winkler, Manitoba, in 1944. She and her husband, Clarence, have two children. Magdalene is a professor of English at the University of Toronto. I met her through my sister Susanna.

I interviewed Magdalene Redekop in her office at the university. Later I read with admiration a short story, "Still Life with Menno." She and her sister Elizabeth had written side-by-side stories about the birth and death of their brother, filtered through adult memory.

Magdalene describes the process of childbirth that results in two adopted children for her. She makes a compelling case that motherhood can be complete even if a woman doesn't go through the act of giving birth herself. She also speaks eloquently about Mennonite culture, particularly as she experienced it as a woman who was unable to bear children.

When you first found out that you were going to receive a child, what were your feelings? Or maybe you want to go back further than that?
Yeah, I think I want to go further back and say what it feels like to think you're pregnant and then not to be pregnant, to say what an educational experience it involves for a woman who gradually confronts the reality of her infertility — particularly in a Mennonite community, where childbirthing is very much a part of what forms a woman's identity, almost *the* central feature. The emotions are very powerful surrounding the desire to give birth, and I

had never had any question but that I wanted to give birth. The infertility story is a long story. All infertility stories are long stories, but while in our society generally infertility is a specific burden for a woman to bear, I think it is a greater burden for a Mennonite woman to bear, because in the Mennonite community there is more nostalgia, more sentimentalization, more romanticizing about the actual experience of childbirth. Why that is I don't exactly know, but I believe it to be a reality of being a woman in a Mennonite community. Perhaps because the less power you have in the structures that there are, the more you emphasize the power you do have, which is to bear a child and to produce that child.

So I had a great desire to bear a child. What I remember particularly is that I had one month in my life when I thought I was pregnant. Many infertile women actually have pregnancies and miscarry repeatedly. There are many different experiences of infertility, but my experience was that I have in fact never been pregnant. But I *thought* I was pregnant. I see it almost as a kind of a mock pregnancy. What had in fact happened is that the fertility drugs I was on had thrown my whole cycle off and actually I had not even ovulated that month, so the reason why I did not have my period was that I had not ovulated. And the result of this was a situation where the signs in my body were miming the signs of pregnancy, which is to say that my breasts swelled up, I was lethargic, I was feeling especially relaxed — especially, you know, cat-like and happy. I certainly felt: this is what it's like to be pregnant! I went to see my doctor and the pregnancy test came back negative. He disagreed with it. He was one of the top infertility specialists in Toronto, I thought, Well, he must know what he's talking about. He said: "All the signs indicate that you are pregnant, and I say you're pregnant." So I went out on clouds, and the next couple of weeks seemed like a very long time because it was so beautiful, I had such a wonderful experience! I read the books on what it was like, I devoured the books. I was, after all, almost forty years old, had always planned to be, and had been trying for a couple of years to get pregnant. I probably know more than any woman I know about how the fetus develops in the first couple of days after conception, all of that. To go into my doctor's office — I had not yet menstruated — at the point when I thought he was going to confirm the diagnosis, and to have him look at my temperature chart and to say, "Oh no, you're not pregnant after all, you can't be" — it was a very, very emotional time, I was very angry with the doctor. It was shattering to have thought that I was pregnant and to not be. But it was an eye opener for me. It was at that point that I confronted the reality of my infertility, and the mockery of this, because I felt as if nature had cheated me. It had played a nasty, nasty trick on me by miming the signs of pregnancy, by catching me up in that. But it also showed me that you could have the emotions without really being pregnant. That's something that's very important for adoption. You can have the emotions without having the biology. I think there's a kind of essentialism in our society generally which is accentuated in a Mennonite community, the romanticizing — you know, the "blood runs thicker than water." We have a strong element of that, which comes from our seclusion. That's all part of what is challenged when you adopt. And it was at that point that I sat down with my husband, we talked about it and we decided: "This is ridiculous, I cannot take this any more, this up and down roller coaster, thinking I'm pregnant, I'm not pregnant." We decided to be constructive, to go about the process of adopting and getting a baby that way. And that's what we did, with very happy results. My children bring me intense joy and satisfaction — that's to make a long story short, that's the happy ending. But in the interim I learned a lot.

Did you tell a lot of people?
Unfortunately I had told several people that I was pregnant. That's always a mistake. The reaction showed me right away how people do not understand adoption, I consider it a sort of profound failure of the imagination in our society of not being able to understand that these are human bonds and social contracts we're talking about that are every bit as intense as the biological ones, if not more so. When you adopt it's very conscious. All the commitments are very conscious. You have to think about whether or not you want to be a parent, and you have to articulate why. At one point when we were having the home studies done, we felt that if everybody had to do this, there would be almost no children born in our society. [laughs] One of my sisters had a nightmare after I phoned to tell her that I was not pregnant and I had to admit how shattered I was. She described only a fragment of it to me. It had something to do with my father holding the baby that had been born of me, and then she broke into tears and she couldn't go on. Clearly in the dream this baby was severely deformed, and she said, "You know, Maggie, this baby was not meant to be. I am sure it was not meant to be." And I said, "But I was not pregnant! I was not really pregnant!" She had constructed a whole horror story surrounding the biological process, which was connected up with the image of the father and with the image of punishment. I always felt that a lot was revealed to me about Mennonite attitudes to reproduction.

Just in your own experience.
Yes. In the experience of adoption and the failure of people to understand what's really involved, and how deep the emotional bond is. Of course it's a challenge, too (the concept of ethnic identity as something you're born with), when you adopt mixed-race children, as I did. I have a daughter who

looks Chinese, and people say, "Will you bring her up Mennonite?" Right? Those kinds of questions wouldn't come up if she didn't look Chinese. So I guess I'm saying it tests, and has tested for me, a lot of attitudes to reproduction, and has made me question the kind of romanticism that surrounds them in a Mennonite community.

Right from square one adoption is a conscious thing, you have to think about whether or not you want to do it, and what that means. I've learned that men generally are more resistant to adoption than women, which is a curious thing. It seems surprising, since the woman carries the baby after all, but it seems to be men, and this also is revealing, I think, of the patriarchal structures of our society. I think it stems from something Freud explores in *Moses and Monotheism* when he says that the reason why we name our children after the male line is that men have to have some evidence that it was their child, that the woman has physical evidence, it came out of my body, but the man doesn't have that, and so the child carries the man's name to show, it has to be legal, there has to be paper work, there has to be a legal connection to give proof of the biological connection. There's something about that that resembles the adoptive mother's experience, because you do the paper work, you make the conscious decision, and it's not biological, and — I don't know, you learn so much about our society's attitude to genealogy. I had always been suspicious of it anyway. In fact, when I was growing up, I think I used to say I would want to have one child by birth and then I would adopt the rest. I wanted to have the experience of childbirth, and I still feel that it's something I've missed. But I don't think it's a very important thing to have missed. I thought to myself at the time when I was infertile, this is something I have to have, I will not have lived fully if I have not experienced childbirth. I now feel that that was the conditioning of the sentimental baggage of Mennonitism and of the patriarchal society we live in generally. That was the most dispensable part of the baggage. Because what I really feel is that I would not have wanted to live without being a mother, and the experience of mothering. One of my friends was very honest, she said to me, "Maggie, the birthing experience is wonderful. But everything that is wonderful about being a mother is what happens after that." And I know people who have both adopted and given birth who say the same thing. It's the day to day. It's the living in the world of wonder that a child creates. It's all of that.

Did you feel you knew a lot about childbirth and pregnancy and family planning when you first got married?

I didn't know a lot. I've written a story, which is about the stillbirth of what would have been my younger brother. I've only just done that a few weeks ago. It shows how (here I am, forty-four years old) I'm just beginning to learn the impact of childbirthing experiences in the family generally. I don't feel I learned a lot of hard education. Of course I went to see a doctor when I got married in 1966. It was late enough so that I got information about birth control and I went on birth control. I knew that in actual fact my mother was probably opposed, but I did not talk to her about it. It was not a subject of conversation. When I found out I was infertile, I knew that many people in the Mennonite community would sort of take that as a punishment from God (that's what you get for having waited so long) or a punishment of nature, or whatever. This is a sort of folklore. Because I am aware of the pain of infertile women, I am aware of the cruelty of the folklore, I'm not saying it's all cruel, but I am aware of that aspect of it, and I feel that what I had was an uninterrogated body of folklore rather than information about pregnancy and childbirth. Because the reality for my mother — my mother had twelve children, sorry, my *parents* had twelve children, my mother had six that lived and two that died — the reality for her (she had very hard labour) was what was true for many women, which was that when you go through childbirth, you go to the gates of death. You risk death every time you create birth. I think we have underestimated the impact of that on women generally. Just because it's not literally true any more, because we now have advanced medicine, it is very rare. As a literary critic, as somebody interested in stories and the impact of myth and fiction, I think we've underestimated it, and I think I had underestimated for myself the fact that my mother almost died each time she gave birth. The last time she gave birth (he would have been my brother Menno, he was stillborn), she was recovering in the hospital and could not attend his funeral. She was close to death. She had one of these, what do they call them, dying experiences. She felt she was dead, she was dying, and she was carried up above. That story, the story of her almost dying, her saying, "Never again will I fear death," the whole association of death with birth was very — I still haven't unpacked the significance of that. With my father's first wife the stories also reinforced that, because she died in childbirth. Her name was Sarah. She gave birth on Christmas Eve, of all things, to a girl, who was called Sarah, and then she died, in convulsions (which ran in the family, we found out afterwards). But that image of death and birth together, and the possible fear that could come out of that I think has been underestimated. For my mother, birth was not easy, she talked about how much she screamed, the stories of her births all blurred into one for me, and it was one long scream.

I wonder if wasn't so painful too because they knew there was no release from it, there was no birth control, and the minute one baby was born all they could face was another one.

I figure my mother and father must have done something, abstinence or something, because she had them every two years, regularly, but then maybe that was just the rhythm of her body.

And she may have breast-fed them.

Yes, she did breast-feed for a long time, so that would have helped. But I think this other point about the punishment aspect: I experienced it not as the actual death of children but the infertility, which is kind of a figurative death of the children you might have had, the children I never had. It's not as if infertility didn't used to be a problem. I remember my mother saying, before I had adopted children (and I adopted children after my mother died, which is one of the sadnesses in my life; it's painful for me even to talk about the fact that she did not live to see my children because she would love them so much), I remember her saying at one point — we were looking out the window at one of the neighbour women, and she was talking about how frustrating, how irritating that woman was, and she said, "Oh dee weet je nich, dee haft noch niemols Tjinja jehaut" — "She knows nothing, she has never had any children." And I said, "But Mother, I have never had children, either." And she said, "Oh but that's different, you're my daughter." But it wasn't different, it was a blow to my — it wasn't even a blow. I mean I knew that that was there, but it was an articulation of something I felt as a constant undercurrent. She became the voice, not just for herself, but for Mennonite society as a whole. If you are a woman and you have no children, you do not know anything, you do not know life, you have not experienced the ultimate. That's what I mean by romanticization.

Do you think Mennonites did it more than others?

I think so, yes. It's heightened among Mennonites — and as I say, there may be a whole variety of reasons for it. I think it has to do partly with being a rural society and the largeness of the family, the family values, so the woman is the one who becomes the vessel, the vehicle for the procreation for the ongoing life, and she is at least acknowledged as having power in that area, and since power is, or was, so radically denied in any other area, you take it where you can get it, right? and that's a very important place to get it.

So obviously it was something that you wanted to experience, so you adopted.

I wanted to experience — well, let's get back to the question you asked me at the very beginning, how did it feel when we first found we were going to have a child, because it might be interesting, given your project, to see how that compares with how it feels when you first find out you're pregnant.

There's a kind of telescoping effect. First of all, we had not waited as long as we had expected to wait, once we actually registered with this private agency. We thought we would wait for a couple of years. In fact I think I was, in the symbolic sense, pregnant less than nine months! All of a sudden — well, we had one loss. There was one child that we were scheduled to get, and we had phoned everybody to say we were getting that child, and then the night before we were supposed to pick the baby up at the hospital, the birth mother changed her mind. We had already named him. We had gone out to celebrate, and then we heard that we weren't getting him. People might be interested to know that an experience like that is like a death. We had not even met this child. We had not seen this child. We had him described. He was part Native Canadian. He had long fingers. I can still visualize a baby boy called Timothy, who was going to be our son. You don't even have to see a child to have the bond. It's like a covenant, a contract that you make, and the emotion that goes with that was very powerful in our case, so we were shattered, and we were in effect in mourning. We had to phone everybody and say, we're not going to commit suicide just because we're not having this baby. And then the social worker said, "Well, we put you at the top of the list for another baby," and that finally did come through.

I don't know what it's like when you have the nine months, but I see friends who are pregnant, and it seems to drag on, for the last couple of months. You seem to be saying, I can't wait for this to happen, because you're waiting and waiting. You are *expecting*. While you expect — we had a particular roller coaster, because the birth mother kept changing her mind, so that when the baby was born (it turned out to be our son Jonathan, at that time he had a different name), he went into a foster home. The birth mother had named him one thing, the foster home people named him another thing, and we, because of our previous experience, didn't name him anything, because we thought, then we'll have another loss, we'll lose another name! [laughs] because we're never going to have a Timothy. It was a real roller coaster, because one day she would say, "I'm going to go in and sign the papers," and the next day she would change her mind, for very real reasons, which I don't want to go into, because it's her private story, but there were legitimate reasons. Women in this position are incredibly courageous. It takes tremendous courage to confront something like this and to do what you think is best for your baby, and she had a really severe struggle. So we were on a roller coaster and just went riding up and down. On the final day of the twenty-one-day period during which the birth mother can change her mind, we were told: "Everything looks like it's going to be alright. Unless she changes her mind today, you can pick up the baby tomorrow." And I suddenly went into overdrive. I went running around buying things to fix up the room. We had a room ready. It was all unnecessary what I was doing, but I went to buy clothes, and it all seemed terribly urgent. It was like a telescoping, an intensification. But I've had other women who were pregnant describe that too. Nesting, I think it's called. So I nested like mad [laughs] on the day before, and then the next morning we got the phone call saying that it was all right, and that we could pick him up, and so we went to the foster home, and — it was an incredibly beautiful experience. The bond was, well it had already happened before we picked him up, I bonded with the piece of paper that said how heavy he was! [laughs] how much hair he had, you know. And the foster parents saying, "He's worth waiting for, he's wonderful, he smiles all the time," etcetera, you know. We bonded with every little detail of information that we got. The bond was very intense indeed, and so that when we picked him up it was, it was — I become inarticulate when I try to explain it, it was so intensely moving.

Your bonding sounds so wonderful, it sounds almost better than it is for women who have given birth and have been under anesthesia.
Exactly. Some parts of it are better. And you don't have postpartum blues! [laughs] So there are some things about it that are better. I wish that I had had — one of the ways of putting what happens to a woman in my position is to say not that I wish that I had given birth, but that I wish that I had given birth to these children. In a way for their sake. It has to do with identity. I guess what I'm saying is that I've crossed a Rubicon or something, I no longer see the need to give birth, the need to have the experience of childbirth as important to my identity, either as a woman or as a Mennonite woman. I feel that it's much more complex, much more related to social constructs, to society, to bonds of contracts. To do a biological essentialism seems to me ridiculous. Sometimes, for the sake of my children (like every mother, I'm protective), I wish I could protect them from the complexities of the struggles of identity which are so much more complex when you are adopted. It isn't that the emotion of the bond between mother and child or father and child is different in adoption. It may be different. It may be more conscious. It may be more intense or whatever, but it's certainly not less. It's not that it's not a mother-child bond. It's that the identity is not the same. Let's say you're a white mother and you have a black child. There's no question that when the child hits adolescence, people are going to comment on him as black, and you do him a disservice if you pretend that there's no difference, in terms of his identity. So in my nostalgic moments I envy the simplicity of the process that other mothers and their children, other fathers and their children go through when their children are theirs by birth and you look like your mother, right? But as I say, that's in my moments of

nostalgia. I don't consider those my best moments. I think that adoption isn't for everyone, but I think infertility was a wonderful preparation for adoption, I think adoption is for mature people, I think adoption is something beautiful and special, which also brings very special rewards, if it's confronted, if it's not denied, it's not something secretive and hush-hush, and I think the final identity that can emerge for the child will be, again, much more conscious. I'm lucky that I have two highly intelligent children, very sensitive children, very funny children. They have a resilience. They'll be able to deal with it. But there's no question that the identity you emerge with, after you're an adolescent if you're adopted, is going to be more conscious, is going to be more resilient, because you won't have some of these myths that I grew up with. So in that sense I feel that it's a special gift to them to be adopted. At the same time — when I feel the closeness with them, the incredible closeness, and I hold my daughter and I say, "How lucky I am to have you as a daughter, I can't believe how lucky," and I love her Chinese eyes — at the same time I wish I could have produced that (not anybody else!) *that* Chinese daughter out of my body. You know, I wish she could have once been one with me, and same with my son, with whom I have a very intense bond also. I wish they could have been one with me once. Partly because it's a story I would like to tell them. But the story that we have written for them necessarily separates the experience of childbirth, which begins with, of course, their birth parents. And we know the birth parents' names. We know enough good things about them so that we can go against the grain of the tendency of our society to put those people down. I think it's very wrong, very bad for adopted children to grow up with a negative view of their birth parents, so we try to convey respect for the birth parents.

Did you feel that there were any links between your mother and your grandmother and you when you became a mother?

Yes, I did. As I suggested earlier, for me that was painful, because both my mother and my grandmother are dead. The continuity which I would like to experience is not there. I have not regretted being a so-called older mother. I'm not saying everybody's a better mother when they're forty, but for me, I think I've been a better mother at forty than I would have been at twenty. But one thing that I really do regret: my mother died when she was only sixty-six, so she could be alive now, and my sisters say to me, "Oh, it's too bad that Mother isn't alive because she would absolutely adore Susanna." And I ask them questions about what she did as a grandmother. I think that if she were alive, her response to my children would be so intense that it would have been an education for her, and it would have brought us closer together in terms of identity. The result of the fact that she is dead, and that we can't do that, means that I — it's made me creative. I end up writing about it, end up constructing ways of trying to heal splits in my own identity, speaking to the ghost of my mother. As far as my grandmothers go, I feel very warmly towards my grandmother on my mother's side. My grandmother on my father's side I never knew, but my grandmother on my mother's side was a very important person, but never so much in that connection. I always thought of her as a wise person, who sat in her rocking chair and told people not to gossip. In some ways she went against some of the feminine excesses. I knew her at a time when she was no longer able to cook. All the stereotypes that I hear from my friends about their grandmothers who bake and who do all this — my grandmother sat in a chair, crippled by rheumatism, and had a wonderfully warm face and an incredibly tolerant attitude to life. "Dee haft uck noch siene goode Sied," she would say — "He will also have his good side" — when people gossiped. She had a kind of wisdom and a kind of oracular quality, sitting there in her rocking chair. My memories of her have very little to do with childbirth, almost nothing to do with childbirth. She's been an important person in my life, partly because my father admired her. I remember that he had great respect for her and for that tolerance, for the fact that she would not enter into the pettiness of gossip that happens in small towns. That's my memory. That's my lasting, enduring memory of her.

What about bonds to other women? Anything to do with motherhood, this shared experience of motherhood?

It's different because I'm a working mother. I feel kind of alienated from the other mothers in the schoolyard and when I go to the Mennonite centre and talk to other Mennonite women. I sometimes feel a distance when people talk about breast-feeding. I feel that there's a glowing romanticism about that. I felt that before, you know, before I even knew I was infertile, I didn't share that, ever, such an intense response to it. I respect it and accept it in other people, but it's not a bond, it's not a basis of my bond. The basis of my bond, I think, to other women, has — I was going to say it's deeper than that, except that sounds arrogant — it has to do with women with whom I can articulate. My bonds with other women are with women like Di Brandt, who has been a mother, who has given birth, but who is articulating her response to the Biblical story which is Father, Son, and Holy Ghost, and where is the mother, right? [laughs] the virgin mother, right? did she scream when she was in labour, you know? like my mother screamed when she was in labour. The sanitizing of the Christian story that has happened: my bonds are with the women who are able to articulate and be honest about their own response, and to be resistant and to question, and so my bonds are on that basis more than with the biological things.

Being a mother, is it a whole experience, does it encompass all of the spiritual, emotional —

Everything I do? Yeah, I think so. Maybe it ought not to, but it does. Everything I have done since I had children involves the children. I have continued to work. I have continued to write. In fact, I have written more, and produced more since I've had children. I'm astonished, I've been far more productive. I don't waste so much time. Some of that is just that you have to stretch your time, you have to organize so much, but it's also that I've been stimulated. I have colleagues, female colleagues, who did not do this, who live more of a bifurcated life. With me it ended up being that I could not continue to function as a teacher and as a scholar if the subject of that was not changed and did not respond in some way to being a mother. So I am a different — I wouldn't be able to say, don't ask me how [laughs] — but I think I am a different kind of a teacher to some extent now than I was before. I'm more playful. I bring in nursery rhymes and use child examples, if nothing else, and certainly my writing and my literary criticism is thoroughly suffused with my concerns about mothering. The book I have written on Alice Munro is about mock mothers [*Mothers and Other Clowns: The Stories of Alice Munro*, Routledge, 1992], and the short story I have just written, "Still Life with Menno" has to do with mothering. Everything I have done since becoming a mother is like a sort of palimpsest, you know, something overlayering the stories of my mothers and of my ancestors who were mothers. I very much feel myself going in that direction, so in a sense my own creativity comes out of watching my own children create, watching the world of wonder that they create around them, and it penetrates every aspect. I think there isn't an aspect of my life that has not been influenced by that.

So in effect you are a very fertile woman after all.

[laughs] Thank you, Kathy! I think so. I've become very fertile since adopting. People say, will you write another story? and I say, well I don't know if I'll have time since I'm so busy with the children and everything, but my imagination is teeming with things I'd like to create, things I'd like to say.

HILDEGARD MARTENS

Hildegard Martens, my husband's sister, was born in Hearst in northern Ontario in 1940, and grew up in Cartwright, Manitoba. She chose to have a baby in 1983. Hildegard was employed by the Province of Ontario's Ministry of Skills Development as a researcher at the time of our interview. She earned her Ph.D. in sociology at the University of Toronto.

Hildegard is a professional woman who heeded her biological clock in time to have a child when she was over forty. The procreative urge and maternal feelings can be so deeply buried that a woman can be quite unconscious that she has them. Then, after they are discovered, there is a nest to be prepared, particularly if the woman is single and has no partner to share the financial load.

I DON'T REMEMBER CHILDBIRTH BEING talked about very much, but I certainly was aware of the whole process of birth, having grown up on the farm. For example, we had a cat that was very affectionately known just as "Kitty" — a very maternal creature, because she produced kittens on a regular basis. This was always very exciting to me — to find a new batch of kittens in the barn — which in turn contributed to my lifelong love of cats.

Also, I witnessed the birth of a calf, which was almost a frightening experience because I saw all the afterbirth and I wasn't quite sure what that was — it had never been explained. I just saw a great big mass of jelly-like substance, all different colours, and I was quickly told to leave the window. Nevertheless, I was fascinated with the behaviour of the animals on the farm.

I don't recall Mother talking about her own births, until years and years later, when I did a tape recording of her, and I asked her specifically about the birth of her children. I remember her talking a little as if having children was a burden. I got that sense because it was associated with the hard work she had to do up north and later on the farm. I believe she had a lot of joy in her babies — that she loved babies. But they also represented hard work and the way she put it, "And then another one came, and I was barely recovering, when I got pregnant *again.*" I remember saying to her, "But Mother, weren't you excited about it?" and she said, "Well, how could I be, because of all the work I had to do?"

When I was growing up I had the impression that her life was very hard and didn't offer a lot of rewards. I grew up thinking it wasn't great to be a woman. I didn't feel that she was encouraging me to get married. She wanted us to make something of ourselves. She would say, for example, "Develop your talents." Dad, too, wanted us to study and read as much as we could. I'm not saying that they said, "Don't get married," they never said that, but I certainly felt that I should choose a lifestyle that was a little easier than theirs.

My mother used to say that I was fascinated with babies as a young child, and whenever I saw one I wanted to hold or touch the baby and I used to say to her that when I grew up, all I wanted to do was to be a mother. Apparently. [laughs] Which is hard to believe in light of the way my life developed. At some point, probably my teenage years, I cut that off somehow. I didn't see very many young children at that stage, although our neighbours had quite young children. I remember visiting them and feeling overwhelmed by their demands.

I began to focus more and more on how I could develop a life that would be more exciting. There were so many adjustments to make, moving from a farm to a city, and not knowing just what to do. After high school I had no firm career plans and at high school the expectations were certainly there that you would have a boyfriend (and I had boyfriends) and that you would marry, probably in your early twenties, and I certainly experienced those expectations. At some level, I wanted that too. At another level, I feared it, because it seemed to represent a hard life and not much fun.

Somewhat like your mother's life, the way it sounded to you!

Yes. [laughs] When I was working, I kept hoping to find a job that I would really like. I was job-oriented even then. I didn't find very good jobs just after high school. With coming from the country, being eighteen and only having grade twelve, you can't get a very exciting job. My first job was with Monarch Life Insurance — I was a mail/posting clerk and it was very frustrating. Then I went to Teachers' College — not something I really wanted but something I did to escape the boredom of my previous job and also because Dad thought it was a good idea. There weren't that many options for women at that time (1958-59).

I remember thinking during my practice teaching, I can't cope with this room full of children. I couldn't imagine having children of my own. Children became less attractive to me in those years. Finally, the opportunity came along for me to go to university. I remember very clearly saying to my sister Ingrid, "But if I decide to go to university, that doesn't mean I won't get married, because I don't want to give that up for a university life. I still want to get married and have a family," but I felt almost apologetic saying that. I felt as though I should make a choice. I really didn't even believe that I could do both — I don't know who I was arguing with, myself probably.

But when I went to university, I just loved it so much and whole worlds opened up — psychology, sociology, history. It was very exciting. I learned a lot of things — certainly my whole belief system was questioned, the one that I held up to then. I had never been a very orthodox Mennonite, but I now began to question things in a different way, and I read Marx and other social philosophers. Marriage took a back seat at that time. The influences of the time — the sixties — were very strong. This was a time when people were experimenting with new ways of being and thinking. I had a boyfriend, but whenever marriage was mentioned, I postponed that notion.

So the years went by. I worked for a couple of years, and then I decided to go on for graduate work, and I came to the University of Toronto in 1969. Again, all thoughts of marriage and having children, whenever they surfaced, were put out of my mind. Because I was now determined to develop a career, and the idea of economic independence became paramount in my mind. And the more that I read, and I read a great deal of feminist literature in the early seventies, the more I felt economic independence was what I really wanted. I began to view marriage as quite oppressive. I kept thinking, Maybe I'll meet someone who will share my views and then marriage will still work out. It wasn't as though I had totally abandoned that idea. But I never seemed to meet just the right person, and it never seemed to work out, probably because most men weren't ready for change at that time. It wasn't until I was in my early thirties that a crisis occurred in my life. Having put my emotions "on the back burner" for so long caught up with me and I realized that there was more to life than books, ideas, and careers. Through some therapy I undertook at the time, I became aware of my longing to have children. This urge was so powerful, it was almost frightening.

I wanted to make my relationships work after that and I tried very hard with some of the men that I met. I broke off a relationship which I knew wasn't leading anywhere. And then I had a series of friendships and relationships that I hoped would work out. The urge to have a child became paramount. Around this time (1977) I received my Ph.D. in sociology.

Finally, I met someone I liked a lot and who valued my independence. I trusted myself to fall in love for the first time in my life and I lived with him for a couple of years. Unfortunately we didn't agree on having children. I felt I had to make a choice: either I stay with him and perhaps never have children, because by this time I was thirty-eight, or leave him and have a child on my own. I had been reading articles about this, where single women found a way to have a child on their own. And it was very, very difficult. I would confront him, he felt very pressured and we both realized that it wouldn't work, and that we'd have to separate.

After that I started to look into ways that I could have a child on my own. The method that I chose was very carefully thought out and planned and, I feel, a very ethical choice on my part. I am proud that I finally found the courage to do it. It wasn't easy to do. I felt very alone. I couldn't ask . . . [her voice breaks] I didn't think that I could broach that subject very easily with members of my family. It was, and still is, a very novel thing to do. It's done, but it's not done frequently, certainly not in "the Mennonite community." I talked it over with a close friend of mine, Edith, your sister. And I think Edith understood my longing, because she certainly feels strongly about children. It wasn't easy for Edith, though, to say, "Yes, go ahead," because she knew what it was like to be a single parent, having been one for a number of years. So she, rightly, didn't want to say too much. And Helga, my sister, didn't think it was a great idea. She'd had some experiences which made her believe that this might be a difficult thing to do. And I didn't think that my mother or my father would be the right people to talk to.

At my age, it was time to take that responsibility for myself, so I went ahead and I really didn't have any encouragement, except from one friend, Joanne, whom I met through the Gestalt Institute of Toronto. I was very lucky to have met her, because whenever I said to people, "I really want a baby more than anything," they would say, "Are you sure you really want that, or is this just a selfish notion, are you acting on the 'me decade' idea, where now you have a career, and the only other thing that you're missing is a child?" I accepted that for awhile, but then I started thinking, Well, for what other reason do people decide to have children? I mean, it's always selfish in the beginning, it's not until the child is there that it can be other than that.

So anyway, Joanne, having lost a child herself and being in her mid-thirties, said to me, "I have decided that I want to have children. I'm not married either and I'm going to find a way." And she said, "If that's what you want, do it. Find a way to do it and forget about what people might say or think!" and I felt, yes, she's right; for one of the first times in my life I'm going to follow my instincts and emotions rather than my head. Because there had been other times, when I would just follow my head and not my heart. So that was good, having her say that. And I'd call her up when I was pregnant and talk to her about whatever doubts I had about being on my own. I saw her as a friend, as well as a therapist, and it was invaluable to have her support.

As I was thinking about doing prenatal classes, I thought, I'm going to be the only woman walking in alone, and there will be all these women with husbands and it will be hard. I told Edith about that and she volunteered to come with me. I was so surprised. I thought, she's going to take an evening out of her busy life to come with me. I was very, very touched by that. Because once I was pregnant, Edith thought it was a great idea, she was very supportive. She came to all my prenatal classes and I read a lot but I was still frightened of the experience. No matter how much I seemed to read, I still wasn't completely relaxed about it. I don't know how to explain that, except — if I go back in my childhood, I know one thing that always haunted me was that I grew up believing that my father's first wife, my oldest brother Henry's mother, had died in childbirth. I had believed that very strongly. There were many pictures which showed my dad holding Henry, standing at her open coffin. It wasn't until years later that I learned she hadn't actually died in childbirth, she had died several weeks later — because of a weak heart, the result of rheumatic fever in childhood. So I don't know if that contributed to this fear; it's quite possible it did.

I didn't get ready for having the baby. I wasn't well organized in the house; it was as though I had a superstition about it. And I asked Helga if she would come to the birth. Helga was "big sister." At times when my mother wasn't available to mother me for whatever reason, when she didn't have the energy or resources or understanding at various times in my life, Helga had often stepped in. The date when Jamie was supposed to arrive was June 5th, so Helga arrived a few days ahead of time. We sat around the house. I was huge [laughs] but there was no sign that I was going to go into labour! So for two weeks we talked about all the things we always used to talk about — psychology, feminism, sociology — very little about this new event that was about to happen. It was as if I was still living in a fantasy world, not really having come to terms with how my life would change. And not daring to think about the birth, almost — Oh, I wish I could go back in time and do it over again! if we could just eliminate the fear and I wouldn't be so frightened now, you know? I'd had doubts in my pregnancy too, about the baby, what and who was he going to be like, and whenever negative feelings would crop up, I'd try not to let them dominate me, because I didn't want to be negative, I was really very happy. I loved being pregnant. I just loved the feel of the kicking inside and I loved the look of my belly — I would often look at myself in the mirror. I felt like I wanted to display it, walk down the street proudly and I did. I really felt complete and whole as a woman.

And very much into your body rather than your mind, eh?
Yes! Just so much! It was like a blossoming for me, that pregnancy. It's just that I'm also the kind of person who worries and who has "negative tapes" inside my head and those would sometimes torment me. And the waiting was actually not that bad, because Helga was here and we talked a lot.

And then finally, we were sitting around a table at my house, and Jeff, a friend of mine, had come over with his daughter, who was about seventeen, and we were playing Trivial Pursuit, and I started to feel some cramps, so I said, "I think this is it." It was far too early to even think about going to the hospital, in retrospect. But I was so nervous and they started getting nervous too, everybody felt maybe I should go, and we went, and nothing happened. The contractions didn't get closer or stronger, they were just more or less the same, and they told me they thought it was a false labour, even though I was two weeks overdue. What happened then, I can't remember — isn't that strange, I can't remember this! I don't remember whether they sent me home or not, but I know that was a false labour.

I spoke to my obstetrician and he said, "If by such and such a time you're not in active labour, I'm going to have to induce the labour, because I'm just a little concerned that we shouldn't wait any longer." I'd had many ultrasounds and they were worried about the amniotic fluid, whether there was an adequate amount of it. I was not too happy about the thought of being induced, because I had read that the contractions were very painful.

So finally the time was set for me and it was eight in the morning. I dreaded that, I didn't feel good about it at all. I felt like I was being wheeled off to something unknown and scary. I had many contraptions strapped on to me — I had a fetal heart monitor and an I.V. The nurse couldn't find my veins; I was extremely bruised. I must have had a catheter, too. I know that I couldn't get up to go to the washroom, there were just a lot of wires attached. The labour room was very, very tiny and both Edith and Helga were there, and they could scarcely turn around in it. I had finally received permission for them to be there and that had taken a bit of doing, because at first the hospital staff weren't keen on having them there but finally they agreed. I think the fact that they were both nurses helped. When the contractions started, they were quite severe. I tried the breathing process but — I don't know whether I didn't have enough faith in myself or what.

So you were induced?

Yes, I was given a pill every so often which would cause a contraction to occur. And around noon I got the epidural. The fetal heart monitor was on all the time. I can remember feeling stressed about it, not really knowing what it said, and when to be concerned. Edith and Helga were watching it, but at times, they seemed to be confused about how the lines should be, and when there might be problems. The nurses would come in and say, "Oh, this isn't working too well, should it be doing that?" Those comments don't exactly help! [laughs] Edith was trying to be very supportive and telling me to breathe. In retrospect, the pain doesn't seem so terrible but at the time it seemed quite severe. I kept expecting it to be worse. I thought that it would get worse and worse — that was what I was afraid of. It was sharp and long, and so it went until I gave birth around ten o'clock that night. What happened was, finally, that the epidural had worn off, and the contractions seemed to be closer together and stronger, and I said, "I need it topped up." And the nurses or the doctor hadn't been in to look at me for a long time. And they didn't come and they didn't come and I kept calling for the anesthetist to come in and top it up. The whole process of getting the epidural is not pleasant either. Because they give it to you in the spine and I had read that if it goes in the wrong place, it can have all kinds of negative consequences. But once you have it in, and it's successful, then having it topped up is not a big deal.

But he didn't come back and finally my doctor said, "Well, I don't think I'll be able to stay, my daughter's graduating tonight. I would have loved to stay to see the baby, but I can't," so he left. I was very disappointed. But he had his assistant there who came and examined me and said, "Well, you're fully dilated!" and at that point I should not have had the epidural topped up. But he thought that I should, he was going along with me. Instead of saying, "I think you can go through this now, you can just push the baby out now," he said, "I want to see how you push." And he said, "I don't think you're going to be able to push this baby out." I was given no confidence in my ability to push the baby out. So they did top it up, and then of course I didn't feel a thing, nothing. And when the time came, apparently I was pushing very well, but he had decided to use low-level forceps. He said that there was evidence of meconium, and that was why he decided that it was time to get the baby out quickly because if they breathe this in it can cause damage. Well at that point I just took his advice, because I wanted the baby to be OK. So he used the low-level forceps, but he told me later he hardly had to use them, that I really was pushing, although I didn't have any sensation at that point.

I wanted to see the baby being born by looking in the little mirror that hung over the delivery table. It kept moving; I kept saying, "Move the mirror so I can see!" But the truth is I never saw the head come out. And it all went very fast then, too, at the end. I remember Edith shouting out, "Oh, he's so cute!" and I started to cry, because of the relief, just knowing that he was OK, that everything was all right, that he seemed to be fine. And — oh! yes the relief, because up to then I hadn't believed, really believed that I would give birth to a normal, healthy baby. And — the feeling! They whisked him away to clear out his lungs, so I didn't have him immediately, and I was aware of them doing that. And then they brought him back and they put him on my breast right away, and I remember this so well, him looking up into my face. He did that right away. His eyes were just seeking my eyes. When I looked into that face, I felt something so powerful, I had never felt in my life. And then he went right to the breast and he sucked like he knew exactly how to suck! He was just beautiful! And I remember calling Mom that night and saying, "I'm so happy!" and I felt that way. I just felt waves of happiness. He was a perfect-looking baby. He had very, very beautiful skin probably because he was overdue. He had beautiful colour already and — whatever doubts I had dissolved totally. I just accepted him 100 percent; he was my baby. And the fact that he was a boy — I had known that because I'd had an amniocentesis — I had initially wanted a girl — just didn't matter at all. I adored him, he was just perfect. I'm looking at pictures right now, taken at the birth — it was a wonderful, wonderful time for me.

I loved breast-feeding, I loved it! I had a little bit of tenderness. I used to put a little salve on the nipple. I breast-fed till he was two and a half and [laughs] as he got older, he used to say things to me, like "Other side!" [laughs] Can you imagine? Sometimes he'd say, "All gone!" And he had his own pet name for nursing, which was "Seddy go." I don't know where that came from, something to do with "Teddy" and not being able to say "Teddy" and coming up with "Seddy" and "go." It was his own little name, and he used to say "Seddy go, seddy go."

At least nobody else knew what it was then!

No! And I used to nurse him in all the places that I could. I got to be quite blasé about it. I'd pick him up — I had stayed home until he was seven and a half months old, which was not long enough — [sighs] I had to go back to work and that was very difficult. Mom stayed for the first three months, and then I had a nanny for awhile. But when I took him to day-care, he was twenty-one months and I was still nursing him then. I used to go pick him up at day-care and the first thing I'd do was nurse him and I did it right in the lobby, I didn't care. Parents would come and go but I just sat there. I had my coat around him and it was such a comforting, wonderful thing to do, for him and me, to connect that way.

If I had not wanted another child, I would have found some way to work part-time but I was motivated to have another child, so I thought I'd better work full-time so that I would have the money and take the pregnancy leave with my second. So I do have some regrets about that, thinking back. I would have wanted to spend more time with him as a baby, an infant — but I did spend every available moment, weekends and evenings. [sighs] I know when I'm an old, old lady, I'm sure I'm going to [laughs] look back on this time as the most wonderful period of my life even though there are some things that I would have liked to have been different — to have been in a more natural environment, to have been more relaxed myself, to have had more encouragement from the medical personnel.

If you could do it over again, knowing what you do now, would you do it differently?
I think I'd do it differently. One thing I would do is work on myself not to be so afraid. I would do more relaxation exercises and be more accepting of the process and even of the pain itself. Not to fight the pain, but to accept that part of it. I don't know if I'd have an epidural or any of that. It's hard to say before you know what the experience is, but now that I *do* know what the experience is, I could say that more clearly. And for younger women, home births, or midwife-assisted births are great. I was over forty. I don't know if it would have been a great idea for me to have had my baby outside of the hospital.

I'm wondering if I'll be the only one in the project who has talked to you about being a single mother by choice.

So far yes! I don't know of anybody else in the Mennonite community, do you?
Not in the Mennonite community. It would be interesting to know if there are any others! I know that I didn't give it a lot of thought [laughs] what the Mennonite community as such would think about it. I certainly thought about reactions of family and friends and I never really heard any negative comments from anybody in the Mennonite community except maybe my

Uncle John. One of Mother's friends in Leamington, Ontario, an eighty-two-year-old man, said, "I think it's just great what Hildegard did! She wanted to have a child and she was able to have a child, financially, and it was the right thing to do."

I know there have been women who have given birth to children on their own, but not by choice.
I mean by choice. And when I say by choice, I don't mean that I wouldn't have preferred to be in a family unit. But I felt time was running out and I didn't want to get married to someone just for the sake of getting married so as to have a child, and maybe that person would not be the right person. I didn't want to make *that* kind of choice.

This is happening to more and more women now. I read about it happening to women who are in their mid- and late thirties — the demands of pursuing a career and a desire for motherhood create a pressure that makes it difficult to find the right mate. The feminist movement has contributed to the emphasis on careers. I still support the views of the feminist movement but there was a bit of an over-emphasis on careers for awhile, that the career was more rewarding than child rearing.

I think motherhood was viewed negatively maybe, too, because in some ways birth practices were at their worst for a while in the fifties and sixties, and birth was not a very rewarding experience. Motherhood had never been highly valued by society, and feminism seemed to pick that up. But now we are redefining that.
The mistake they made was to say that women should have everything that men have and that seemed to mean that you should succeed primarily at a career. And if that meant that you didn't get married and didn't have children, that was OK. Women should be able to make the choice to be childless but sometimes they did it without a clear awareness of their own needs and desires. They made the choice not to have children because they thought that was the only way to be successful, to be recognized and to have respect in society.

I much prefer the newer way, but now there's a danger of society having too great expectations of what women's roles should be. Now we should be everything, we should have careers, *and* we should be very good at them *and* we should aim high. We should be lawyers, we should be doctors, we should be executives *and* we should be mothers and wives *and* we should do all those things well. A superwoman syndrome, in other words. A lot of women are feeling it. There has to be a clearer understanding of the roles and responsibilities of men and women and more sharing between the sexes.

And the workplace — I feel very strongly about this — the workplace is still largely designed according to the traditional family model, where the men "earn the bread" and the women "mind the home." The working hours are most often from nine to five, with overtime and early breakfast meetings expected — this doesn't fit into a schedule where you have small children, they can be sick and you don't see them for long periods of time. This is one of my frustrations now. I don't see my son enough. By the time I get home, it's late and I can barely make supper and then he has to go to bed. In Sweden they've reduced the working day for parents of young children by two hours. That is recognizing the family as a real unit in society.

And yet in our society it's always seen as a sort of a sop to women. They don't recognize that it would be good for men and *women to see their children more.*
Yes, exactly. So we have a long way to go. We've moved from the traditional model of the family — which was not very successful — to the splintering of the family and to the career women syndrome, where many women were choosing not to get married at all to the super woman syndrome. We have to evolve further!

I wanted to go back to your mother's reaction, once Jamie was born.
Oh, 100 percent acceptance of Jamie! She's been very kind and supportive to me and has stayed with me part of every winter since Jamie was born to help in the house. Mother would not come out and tell me that she supported my decision but I've heard her defend me when she feels that I've been criticized. And I know she loves Jamie very much. It would be difficult for her to come right out and say, "I think you did the right thing." Because in her world, that just wasn't done. The idea of a woman being single and having a child was considered a disgrace at one time. And it must be very difficult to move from that view to a view that is fully accepting of it. It would be nice if she would say that, but I don't know if I have those expectations of her any more. I'm just very glad that she fully accepted Jamie and that we have a good relationship.

I have a lot of regret that my father didn't know about it and that he didn't know Jamie. I think that he would have loved him as well and it would have meant a lot to me to have Dad know about it. He was dying of cancer when I got pregnant and that was hard, you see, because when I was pregnant, I was feeling the joy of my own new developing life. And I wanted to tell him, but I couldn't because it didn't seem like the right time. But sometimes I fantasize about having told him and — I think he would have accepted it very well.

ROBERTA LOUGHRIN

Roberta (Peters) Loughrin was born in Steinbach, Manitoba, in 1966. She and her husband, Tim, have two children. At the time of the interview she was expecting her second baby and was a full-time homemaker.

It was December and my year was almost over. I had met Roberta, the youngest mother on the list, at a meeting of the Home Birth Network in Winnipeg. Roberta describes her first childbirth in a hospital. She wanted to have her second baby at home with a midwife, but was also seeing a doctor just in case. Roberta was young enough to be my daughter, which made me feel like hugging her, she seemed so vulnerable. I also realized that she was becoming a mother at the same age as matriarchs like Maria Reimer had done sixty years before. If I try to imagine Maria Reimer at the time of her first birth giving, the image of Roberta comes to mind. If only the wisdom of a woman of Maria's age were always there to draw upon when young women enter the hospital to give birth!

After her second baby was born, I visited Roberta to give her a copy of the tape we had made. She had gone into labour at home with her lay midwife in attendance but decided later to enter the hospital and gave birth there. Going to the hospital was not a failure; it was her decision, and her labour was well advanced when she went in.

I HAD NATALIE LAST YEAR, just after Christmas, and I found out I was pregnant in early May, so I'd been pregnant for a while. I had gone out to Ontario to visit my husband's family, and I had gotten very carsick in the car, and my mother-in-law predicted I was pregnant, and sure enough, she was right. That was a very exhilarating feeling, when I found out. We had said after we got married that we'd leave it in the Lord's hands, when He thought we'd be ready to have children, so six months later I guess He thought we were ready. Little did we know how that would change our lives. And then we thought about a doctor, and we chose one, we heard that he was a Christian, and we liked that, and that he had a very good bedside manner, so that was enough for us. So we had seen him, and gone to prenatal classes — my husband was in long-distance trucking, so he missed about half of them. I did a fair amount of reading, on natural birth mostly, and had anticipated having a natural birth. Then my blood pressure during the pregnancy skyrocketed, I also gained a lot of weight, I gained approximately sixty pounds, so during the last couple of weeks, my doctor was worried that I'd had a precondition of pre-eclampsia, which developed into toxemia, and so I just took his word for all that, very trusting in my doctor, not taking responsibility for looking into things myself. I wish that I would have. But we live and learn.

Natalie's due date was on Christmas day, and we had gone in to see him for a check-up on Christmas day in the hospital in Steinbach, and he was leaving for holidays the next day. Because of the high blood pressure and pre-eclampsia, he said he wanted me to go to Winnipeg to have the baby. He said, "Tonight you'll go into hospital, and you'll have a baby probably tomorrow," and it was very exciting in one way knowing that soon we would have our child, we'd been waiting for so long, but it was very scary, because you get to know a doctor, and you trust in him, all of a sudden you're left in the care of strangers. So three hours later we packed our bags and drove to the city and checked in, and because I was a so-called high risk patient, I had no birthing room, where you go in the beginning and you stay the whole time, and you birth there later on. I didn't have that privilege, and so I was in this little room. Then they put a [prostaglandin suppository] in the vagina, to ripen the cervix so it's ready for labour. So to this day I do not know what a natural labour is. Being induced is very unnatural, it's very quick, it's very painful.

So that was Christmas night, and my husband was there, that was comforting. I got to go to bed around two o'clock. One thing I wasn't too thrilled with was, during that time in that room, on the fetal monitor, an intern came in and wanted to check me internally, and I felt very offended by that. It felt very undignified, I felt more like a slab of meat that was being used as a study piece than like a person. Especially your first time with birth, it's overwhelming.

Why did they have to do that, or do they just want to do it?

They just want to. He came in, and then luckily I looked at my husband, and he knew, just looking at me, that this was not exactly what I wanted, so the nurse came in, and then after that I didn't have any interns bother with me. But with the nurses coming in all the time and checking you out, it's not very relaxing. One nurse was actually very sweet. My back was sore from lying there for a couple of hours, so I had brought a tennis ball to rub on my back, and she noticed that I was about to do this, and she came and rubbed my back and talked to me, so she was actually very comforting. I went to bed at two in the morning and they woke me about eight, or maybe seven, so it wasn't much of a sleep. I was very tired, and then they started to induce me, and then later on they broke my water. Nothing was really happening until about eleven o'clock, I had an enema, and that just started the whole thing, an hour after that everything was on the roll. I would compare it to what I had thought transition stage was going to be like, what I'd learned in prenatal class. It was no gradual onset, it was all of a sudden, back to back, hard labour, and it was just overwhelming. It was very scary and very out of control, I was in a lot of pain. And then they had the fetal monitor going, which would squeeze your arm every ten or fifteen minutes, you can hardly relax with this thing cutting off your circulation, making all these noises, and people fussing over you.

You were always lying down?

Always lying down, I was never allowed to move, except the one time that I went to the bathroom to empty my bladder, that was the only time I moved. So I was not comfortable. The labour had started around twelve noon, and by three o'clock I was screaming for an epidural, and the doctor that was supposed to give it was busy doing surgery or something, so I had to wait. I was ready to be shot in the head. [laughs] I cannot explain the pain, it was very painful. And then I had an epidural, and again, that's a risky thing, but that numbed the pain, and I had a very good sleep after that. I guess I slept for at least six hours. I woke up in the evening sometime, around eightish, and I was almost fully dilated, and then around 9:30 I had the urge to push. The epidural had worn off, so then I could feel the pain once again. It wasn't as extreme, I could actually handle that more than I could handle the pain that had happened earlier.

So at that point I was very excited, even though I was tired and drained, because I knew that the end was soon to come. They took me into the delivery room, and it was again not what I had wanted, bright lights, it looked like you were going into an operation or something, it was certainly not at all what I wanted for my birth, and then they transferred me over to the operation table, so narrow too, you're so uncomfortable, stirrups, the whole bit. I had a nice nurse at that time. And so then she had me starting to push, so I did that for about an hour. And then the doctor came in, whom I'd never met before, and he said I had a couple of pushes left. I was watching in the mirror, and it was exciting. I was feeling very very sick, I guess with all the drugs, and the fatigue, and my body was just — so I told my husband, I'm going to — I am going to — puke! — Oh no, you're not! I ended up puking all over him! [laughs] Yeah, as soon as Natalie came into this world, I — everyone was all excited, and here I was, sick!

My husband was very excited. It was a real joy watching the expressions on his face. So Natalie was born, and they let her on my tummy for just a little bit, and then right away they washed her up, and the nurse and my husband were back in the corner, cleaning her up, and doing whatever they do. And all of a sudden I was in pain again, and I looked down, and there was the doctor ripping out my placenta. Like immediately after the birth, not minutes after, immediately after. And my husband came back and looked, and he just couldn't believe it, he thought he was ripping out my stomach, he was quite grossed out at the whole thing. I thought that was very insensitive of him. I felt everything was so rush, rush, rush, next labour, next woman, get her in. I was quite offended by that.

I got into the recovery room, and they let me nurse Natalie a little bit, but I was woozy. I didn't feel that much bonding with her, I just felt everything was so rushed, and so systematic, it just didn't seem as cozy as I wanted. I was a bit sad, actually. And my husband had gone with the baby; he actually spent more time with her those first hours than I had.

I wanted to recover in Steinbach, because my family and friends were there, so I requested a discharge that morning — if I had known what was ahead of me, I would have just gone straight home, but I didn't. When we arrived at the Steinbach hospital, they hadn't even been expecting us, the city hospital had not even clued them in, so I had to wait there in the foyer. She was the only baby in the hospital, and she had to go in the hallway, she couldn't go in the nursery, and right away I felt like we were kind of aliens. I had a room to myself, and I requested that Natalie be with me, I wanted to nurse her, but they kept giving her the bottles, the sugar water, and fed her, so she wasn't nursing the way she should have been. So that was a real struggle, that first week. I was very unrelaxed, I felt like I was put in jail, I was there for five whole days, which was a very long stay, I didn't have a C-section or anything. And I didn't find the nurses very supportive at all. Natalie had become colicky, she screamed around the clock in the hospital. I was quite uptight, and I wanted so much to bond with her and be close to her, it was overwhelming, because she was screaming, and I was trying to nurse, and she wouldn't nurse, and the nurses were trying to tell me, well, just give up and give her the bottle. I had gone to La Leche League meetings, I was very much aware of nursing, and the benefits, and I wanted this for me and my child. My husband was beside me in all this, he knew how much it meant to me to nurse this child. We were very lucky because my aunt is the one who had started the chapter of La Leche League in this area, so she came, and she gave me some advice. But I knew I needed more support because I wasn't getting it from the nursing staff. It was only when we got home the next day that my milk let down, when there was no intervention of anyone giving bottles, there was no stress involved, I could relax and then nursing started. I had never had any experience with children under about the age of three, I only have a younger brother who's four years younger, I have no relatives, I never babysat, so I had never changed a diaper. I was doing this on faith, and my motherly instincts.

In the hospital they were trying to teach me how to bathe a baby upside down, head first, and I was not comfortable with that at all. I didn't know how to fold a receiving blanket properly, and so I'd ask the doctor to show me. Then the day that I thought I was going to go home, three days afterwards, the doctor had said, "Well, I think we should leave you in, the nurses say you're not quite informed with some of the things, caring of the child, bathing." I felt so hurt, I just cried and cried in my husband's arms, I said, "I'm a mom, I know I'm not perfect, but I've a desire to know, I'm a good mom." The next two days were like an eternity, I just wanted out of there, can I run out with my baby? The last night, I'd finally gotten her to relax around one o'clock, and I put her in the basket right next to my bed, and I was so comforted just having her there. And then out of the corner of the eye I saw a nurse tiptoe into the room. She was about to roll the baby out, and I put my hand on the cart, and I said, "No way, this is my child, she's staying right here." And she said, "I'm sorry, it's against regulations." So we were having this squabble, I told her I was the mother, and I was responsible, and she said, no, I'm the nurse, I'm responsible. And oh, just — get me out of this place! And so she took the baby, and then again I was totally unrelaxed, and I cried the next three hours. And nobody could hold Natalie, just me and my husband, it was just awful.

We got home on New Year's Eve. My sister-in-law had been out, and she had helped Tim clean the house, so it was a very nice welcoming, and things started to relax. Natalie was actually colicky for three months, but I was at home with my family, and alone with my baby, and so I could finally relax. I have nothing good to say about the hospital, except the food. I looked forward to the meals, that was *it*.

So then mothering began for me, and I had this colicky child, and I really had no support on the outside, because my mom was teaching, and my mother-in-law was in Ottawa, and I had no sisters, all my friends had children of their own. My husband went into long-distance truck driving a week after that, and so I was burdened with this baby that screamed all the time. I was thinking, What am I doing wrong, I tried everything, I called people, and I was reading. Finally I was getting very run down and I didn't know what I would do emotionally, I didn't know how I was going to make it through this, I wasn't sleeping, my nerves were shot, and I wasn't eating. I lost forty pounds that first month, I was too weak to even make anything nourishing for myself, so I guess because of that my milk supply was very weak, and about the sixth week, she didn't seem interested in nursing, she cried and cried, and she wouldn't come to me. I tried everything, I called the La Leche League, and a woman from there came and spent a whole afternoon watching me and the baby, worked with me for a couple of days, and said that there was a very slim chance that Natalie would go back to nursing. So I was glad to have that support, and I went back to bottle feeding. And after that the colic soon stopped.

But then my emotions — I don't know what you would want to label this under, postpartum blues, or pre-pregnant [laughs] blues, or having a colicky baby for three months, my nerves just finally went. It was intense and dramatic and scary. My husband had quit trucking, he realized that I needed some help at home, and he had gone into car sales, so that was a real benefit, having him there. I was out of touch with my emotions, I didn't know what was happening to me, and also being a born-again Christian, spiritually speaking, I was really seeking the Lord. I felt very guilty, what had I done wrong, where is the "joy of the Lord is your strength," it's not here! I was very confused, and was seeking help. I went to my physician and mentioned that my emotions were unpredictable and scary, and he right away wanted to put me on an anti-depressant pill. I didn't really want to rely on medication, I wanted to rely on the Lord and myself, and see myself through this. So I got home and thought about it, prayed about it a lot, and I guess being in such a weak state, I said OK; he had said they were non-addictive, so I started taking these pills, and they were so strong that instead of being depressed, I slept all the time, I could not lift my head off the pillow, and I had this four-month-old child to care for. I was sick, I was nauseous, I felt like I had the flu all the time. They said it would get better after two or three weeks, but by that time I said, I'm going to throw these out the window!

I had had one period during this whole time. They had told me that this medication might not bring on the menstrual cycle, so I didn't think that I could be pregnant. Although two months prior to that I still hadn't had one, and my doctor had said, "Oh, maybe you're pregnant," but he never looked into it. It would have been a very easy test instead of having to go on this. Then we found out that sure enough, I was pregnant again. So I got pregnant in March, three months after Natalie was born. My body had gone through a lot. I was starting to lose more confidence in him, and when I found out I was pregnant with this baby, my first reaction was, oh my goodness, how can I be pregnant, I'm having such a hard time just managing right now with my first child, sure I love her, but — another one?! it was overwhelming. I cried at first, and then we went for a car ride, my husband and I, and I said, so many people in this world would do anything to have a healthy child, have been trying for years and years and years, this is definitely of the Lord, we certainly weren't trying. So then I started to accept it.

Two months prior to this a friend of mine had had a home birth, and I was very curious about that. I asked her about it, and I said I'd like to explore that avenue. I contacted a midwife in the area, and she gave me some reading material. I was hesitant at that point on home birth, so I kept reading, and the more I read, the more peace I had. I was so excited, I'd keep going to my husband, "Oh, this is so exciting!" And it felt so good because I was really looking forward to this baby, like oh wow! To me it was like a healing, thinking of a healing process about to occur for the void that I felt with Natalie's birth.

KARIN DIRKS

Karin (Wieler) Dirks was born in Altona, Manitoba, in 1928. She and her husband, Wally, had two children. Karin was a full-time homemaker and a very active volunteer. She died in 1994.

Karin was my last interview in 1988. She was a volunteer with Mennonite Books, a Mennonite mail-order book club, and we were discussing books when she asked me what I was busy with. When I told her, she asked, "Why haven't you interviewed me? I have the happiest birth stories you have ever heard." How could I resist that? Her interview is sprinkled with German expressions, and in one case Karin uses her own hybrid of Germanized Plautdietsch, Zurechtmacher *("rightmaker", meaning bone setter). Karin paid me a compliment: "I did all the work; you hardly said anything, but I had the feeling you listened to every word I said."*

I WAS A SUNDAY BABY, which they say is special. My mother was thirty-three when she married my father, who was a widower. He had three children, and they were quite a bit older than me. My dad must have been about forty-four or so when they married. After they were married three years, I was born, and they were delighted. My dad was a real *Kinderfreund*, he loved babies. So this baby arrived early, and I was actually born in our living room, on a sort of hide-a-bed, I guess, davenport type of thing, and because I came early, there was no preparation, and the doctor was mostly concerned with my mother. I was so tiny when I was born — they say I wasn't four pounds — he didn't even worry about me, he was just concerned about my mother, didn't think I would survive. My father and a Mrs. Rempel, Mrs. Schmidt Rempel, her husband was the smithy down the street, she came to help. My dad said they put me in hot water and cold water and they were trying to revive me and I revived! I guess I started to cry, and they put me in this basket with a hot water bottle, and I survived. And the next morning Dr. Breitenbach came to visit my mother to see how she was, and as he walked in, he said to my dad, "Lebt sie noch?" ("Is she still alive?"), meaning me, and my dad said yes. And he said that was the first time he actually took an interest. So he looked down into this basket to see this thing that was [laughs] alive. My mother said I must have been colicky or what, because for six months I screamed, and I don't think she had enough milk for me. And my father, she said, because I was so little, and he had wonderful hands, because he was a *Zurechtmacher* (bone setter), he would bathe me. She never bathed me I think for six months. She said he would do it, and then he would wrap me in a blanket. You never could make a living with just being a *Zurechtmacher*, so he had a little butcher shop across the street from where we lived, and my mother said he would wrap me in this towel or blanket, and because it was summer, he would walk across the street and weigh me on his butcher scale [laughs] to see if I was gaining any weight. My mother and dad were always so proud, here I grew up to be this tall person — I'm five feet eight and a half inches — from this little thing. And my mother was a very short lady, my father was tall, all the Wielers are tall, so I took after him, but she was always very proud of this fact that I had been so little and so scrawny, and here I grew up to be tall. Although I seem to have caught every childhood disease there was, and I always was deathly ill with them. Maybe there was a lot of hovering over this child, you know, my mother's only one, she never had any other children.

I liked the story of your mother's arrival here. Could you tell that here?
Sure! It's so romantic, I love the story myself. My dad said that when a new influx of immigrants came, they always went to the station to see who might be arriving, maybe it would be someone they knew. This was in Altona. My mother's mother came with her daughters. They had stopped in Southampton, they had a little money, and they bought some very nice hats, so they all had a beautiful hat for their arrival, she didn't want them to look too bedraggled. When they stepped off the train, my mother must have really impressed my father, because he fell in love with her, first sight, just stepping off the train! He thought, Oh, if she's available, that's the one

for me! He'd been a widower five years and he was ready to find a mate. Anyway, turned out that my mother was single, a spinster of thirty-two, and he courted her that winter, and the following year he married her, in 1925. They were married on the farm of *Ältester* (Elder) Johann Klassen, who lived in Starbuck along the La Salle River. They had a nice farm and a lovely woods near the water. And all this entourage came from Altona for the wedding. The ceremony itself was inside at the Klassens', but the *Faspa* (lunch) was outside, as a picnic. My mother wore a white dress and a veil and a *Kranz* (wreath) with the *Myrten* (myrtle). She was always a little bit embarrassed [laughs] about this wedding feast, but on the pictures — we have two snapshots — it looks quite nice: these big white tablecloths on the lawn, and all these people lounging around them, just like on those pictures from Russia, they all seem to have these poses, they loved these poses, [laughs] you know, and they're all around these two huge white tablecloths.

Why was she embarrassed? I don't quite understand.
I don't know. I know when her oldest sister got married in Russia, it was still the good times, and they had this gorgeous *Gut* (estate), which was decorated. My mother said they had this *großer Saal* (large living room), and the *Saal* had these columns, she said, with ivy entwined, and roses and champagne, and the meal was something else, they had it prepared by the Russian cook, it must have been very beautiful, a three-day event! *Polterabend* (evening of gift-giving) and all that! And here she had this meagre little wedding, they were so poor, they had nothing. There's a picture of my dad and her that was taken with a little Kodak camera, I guess, and they're squinting in the sun. She never liked it either. [laughs] I'm sure the young kids now would think that was neat, having a picnic. But in 1925 I guess it wasn't quite the accepted way of having your wedding.

Well, let's turn to your life, and since you're going to talk about the birth of your children, maybe we should talk about you getting married first.
I met my husband in our church. Can you imagine, what a nice place to meet, eh? [laughs] Our church was First Mennonite, this must have been about 1949. Our choir had invited all the university students to come for an evening and we had a program and served lunch. Wally had already graduated, but he came with a friend. We sort of started to talk, and the next thing we knew, I went to a symphony concert with him — that was our first date. We didn't have any money, so we went to the art gallery, and we bicycled and did things like that. We were married in '51, and nine months later Christopher was born. He was conceived on our honeymoon. I didn't think it was possible that you could have a baby [laughs] just that

quickly, you know! And I *loved* babies, I was like my father, *loved* babies. Never had a little younger brother or sister, so I was delighted! I think my mother was somewhat shocked, so soon, you know! but I was just delighted.

I developed toxemia with my first child, so I had to be careful, my blood pressure went up, and so one day Dr. Gunther said, "Well, Karin, I think you're going to have to come in and have your baby." And I said, "Oh, no! I want to wake up in the middle of the night, and say, ohhh, I think this is it, I think maybe now — But if you say I have to go in tomorrow, that's like going for your appendix!" And he said, "All right, you go back home, but take it easy for a whole week, just lie around, don't do anything, and maybe you'll be all right." So I did, and the following week I went in and he said, "No, it's too dangerous for you and for the baby, you better come in." That was about eight days before the due date, so it wasn't that bad. So I went in the following day, and they did a surgical induction, and nothing happened. By about four o'clock I got some pains, and then they were very severe. I didn't go through hours and hours of labour. Wally left about four o'clock, and ten minutes after seven the baby was born. And it was so wonderful. That birth was just — I'll never forget it as long as I live, it was the most exciting thing. I felt very spiritual, I felt that God and I were now making this — I mean it had been created, but somehow, I don't know, I felt very close. Dr. Gunther was there guiding, and he'd say to push, and I'd push, and he said, "There's the head." Well! I went ecstatic! "That's it?!" He said, "That's it." I said, "This is really it?!" He said, "This is it, Karin." I said, "This is *wonderful!* This is what I'm *made* for!" It was so terrific. He said, "Now here comes one shoulder, here comes the other," and then — the baby was born, and it was just — so marvellous, and he picked up the baby, and the baby cried, and I said, "Oh, slap him again, I want to hear him again!" [laughs] That was just something else. And at that time there wasn't too much natural childbirth. I don't think the birth was totally natural, I think I got a little whiff of something, but — oh, I was so aware of everything! Dr. Gunther went down to tell Wally that he had a son, and he said, "Karin is in seventh heaven, she wants to shout this from the rooftops! [laughs] she's ready to climb the Health Science Centre" — it was at the Women's Pavilion. I was really thrilled.

With the second child, I woke up in the morning, five or six o'clock, thinking this was it, and it was. We dropped Christopher off at my mother's about seven o'clock, and then we went again to the Pavilion. I wanted it to be the same, but it wasn't, there was more pain, and I was I think too eager to birth it, I think I used up a lot of energy pushing when I wasn't ready. But it was terrific, too, it was wonderful. And I remember when Dr. Gunther said, "Here comes the head, Karin, it's a little blonde one! I think it's a little blonde girl!" [laughs] But when all of him came out, it was a little boy, and I was delighted! I couldn't have been more happy. It was just lovely.

Did you enjoy the children when they were babies?
Loved them! I really loved them very much as little babies. Wally went on the road just as Tim was born, so he was away a great deal. He went out on the road every week. That became quite a strain eventually. I was very conscientious as a mother, and shouldn't have been. I was hard on myself, but I always said to myself, I never ever want to grow old and say that I didn't play with my children enough. *Never* did I want to say that. For me those years were so important. I mean, I was delighted when they got to school, too, that these stages were reached. But I did enjoy them very much as babies, and as toddlers. Then of course there are things like training, that was difficult, because I had a lot of pressure — my aunts were the kind that trained their children by one year, and —

Yeah, that used to be a real problem between the generations, didn't it?
Oh, yeah, was it ever! And you felt like there was something the matter with you if you couldn't have them trained by a year! So I tried, too. And with boys. Now they don't try, my grandgirls — I have three grandgirls — sheesh! they don't start till they're year two, and then it's *hatzeplatz* (bingo!), it's done. We would drag this out, and put pressure on those little tykes.

I guess they did it because laundry was a much bigger problem.
Well, I had to do them, too, but we did have the hot water, the washers with the wringers, and the whole bit was easier. I did get an automatic washer and dryer when Tim was about two, but during all the infancy I had to do diapers. And you were very proud to hang out these brilliant white diapers on the line! And they had to freeze, because that made them whiter, and then you had this clothes horse when it got too cold to hang them on the line, and they froze on it, then you dragged that in, and — aahh! But anyway, here I am, the mother of two wonderful sons, who have been just marvellous boys.They were very rambunctious as children. I wondered — *huch!* — how's it ever going to be when they're teeners! But I think they got it all out when they were charging around.

Did you nurse your babies? Did you have support from your family?
Christopher I didn't nurse long, because it wasn't fashionable, so after about three months, I didn't. But with Tim, he didn't take a bottle. The other one, if I left, I would leave a bottle for him. But Timmy refused the bottle, he just wanted to be breast-fed, which I did and loved. When we went out in

the evening, I would put him to bed at seven — he was about two months old — and I knew he would never wake up until seven in the morning. He slept very well, so that I could go out and not have to worry about a bottle. I nursed him for six months, and you know why I stopped nursing? Because his father said, "Look, Karin, that kid could be eating raw beef steak, and you're still nursing!" [laughs] So that sort of made me stop! And the poor — I think it was hard on him, because he was still attached to me, he didn't like the bottle. It was a little young to go on the cup at that age.

I get the impression you always look on the bright side, Karin.
Somehow I do, but I also have inner resources, I have inner strengths that I feel I can count on. Don't think that I didn't have birth pains! But I remember thinking, my mother went through this when I was born, my grandmother must have gone through this, it's hard for every mother, and they did it, and I'll do it, I can do it. I hung on to the bed, I really hung on with all my strength. With my second child the nurse thought it was going to be a long time yet, and I said, "Well if you're waiting to hear me make any sounds, or screaming, you won't. So I might be ready and you won't think so, because I won't let out anything." I have such a high threshold for pain.

You considered it sort of work.
Yes! It was all part of the birthing. It can't be the same for everyone, but that's how I am. And I'll tell you, Kathy, when I was giving birth, I thought, maybe this is how dying is. Maybe this is how it is, you're afraid of childbirth, you haven't had it before, all you hear is pain and agony, and how they just want to be out of it, so that they're not aware — and that's the best part! I mean, why get knocked out for that? The labour is hard, but the birthing is so marvellous, and I think, Well, maybe that's how death is, maybe that'll be the best part! Although, I mean, I'm afraid of dying —

It's letting go, isn't it.
Yeah, I don't know. What I'm sort of afraid of is that transition, but I think, I wonder how that is. And then I think, well you didn't know how it would be with giving birth, and it was marvellous! And maybe that's how that'll be.

I've thought about that, too, that birth and dying are probably very much alike. One your head is coming down, and the other, your spirit is leaving through your head, maybe.
But something leaves, yes. — And being this child of older parents, not having any siblings, I was very much loved by my parents. My dad was one

of the younger of eleven children in his family, so when I came along, I had a lot of love from the whole family, they always called me *unser kleines Kusinchen* (our little cousin) — although I wasn't so *klein*, as you know! But I was the youngest, and I always felt very much loved, I felt special. And I always felt that I was special to God, as a kid.

Because you had almost died.
Maybe that's it! I don't know, I've never thought of it in those terms! And I'm blessed with so many friends, I love people, and it just pays off, I think. And if you can express that, too, I mean — gee, you know, I'm no great intelligence or anything like that, but —

It comes from within.
Yeah, my mother often said that you had to have *Mutterwitz,* it was very important to have *Mutterwitz.* I think it's common sense! She'd say *Mutterwitz.* You went a long way on *Mutterwitz*, that means you can apply yourself, and you don't have to be educated for it, it's something that's inborn, your mother has given it to you, as has her mother to her, and so that's my story.

Selected Sources

Angugaliaq, Martha. Recollections of Martha Angugatiaq, Ungalaaq-Inuit Cultural Institute Autobiography Series, Eskimo Point, NWT, Canada X0C 0E0, 1985.

Arms, Suzanne. *Immaculate Deception: A New Look at Women and Childbirth in America.* Boston: Houghton and Mifflin, 1975.

Armstrong, Penny, and Sheryl Feldman. *A Midwife's Story.* New York: Random House Ballantine Books, 1988.

Ashford, Janet Isaacs, ed. *Birth Stories: The Experience Remembered.* Trumansberg, N.Y.: The Crossing Road Press, 1984.

Barrington, Eleanor. *Midwifery is Catching.* Toronto: NC Press Ltd., 1985.

Basham, Ardythe. "Childbirth Options and Services in Winnipeg, A Consumers Guide." Unpublished paper, 1987.

Birch, Darlene. Videotape of a home birth, Winnipeg, Manitoba, 1991.

Blackman, Margaret B. *During My Time: Florence Edenshaw Davidson, A Haida Woman.* Seattle: University of Washington Press; Vancouver: Douglas and McIntyre, 1982.

Brandt, Di. *Wild Mother Dancing: Maternal Narrative in Canadian Literature.* Winnipeg: University of Manitoba Press, 1993.

Burtch, Brian. *Trials of Labour: The Re-emergence of Midwifery.* Montreal: McGill-Queen's University Press, 1994.

Canadian Medical Association. "Obstetrics '87: A Report of the CMA on Obstetrical Care in Canada, 1987."

Carpenter, Carole H. "Tales Women Tell: The Function of Birth Experience Narratives." *Canadian Folklore Canadien, Journal of the Folklore Studies Association of Canada* 7, nos. 1-2 (1985).

Chamberlain, David B. *Babies Remember Birth and Other Extraordinary Scientific Discoveries about the Mind and Personality of Your Newborn.* Los Angeles: New York, St. Martin's Press Jeremy P. Tarcher, 1988.

Davis-Floyd, Robbie E. *Birth as an American Rite of Passage.* Berkeley: University of California Press, 1992.

Duden, Barbara. *Disembodying Women: Perspectives on Pregnancy and the Unborn.* Cambridge, Mass.: Harvard University Press, 1993.

Duerk, Judith. *A Circle of Stones: A Woman's Journey to Herself.* San Diego, California: Lura Media, 1989.

Ehrenreich, Barbara, and Deidre English. *Witches, Midwives, and Nurses. A History of Women Healers.* Old Westbury, N.Y.: The Feminist Press, 1973.

______. *For Her Own Good: 150 Years of the Experts' Advice to Women.* Garden City, N.Y.: Anchor Press, 1978.

Epp, Frank H. *Mennonite Exodus.* Altona, Manitoba: D.W. Friesen, for Canadian Mennonite Relief and Immigration Council, 1962.

Freud, Sigmund. *Moses and Monotheism.* Translated from German by Katherine Jones. New York: Vintage Books, 1939.

Gaskin, Ina. *Spiritual Midwifery.* Summertown, TN 38483: The Book Publishing Company, 1977, 1980, 1990.

Gluck, Sherna Berger, and Daphne Patai, eds. *Women's Words: The Feminist Practice of Oral History.* New York and London: Routledge, 1991.

Handziuk, Debra Gayle. "The Climate for Disclosure: An Examination of Sexual Abuse among Rural Mennonite Families." M.A. thesis, University of Manitoba, 1993.

Harper, Barbara. *Gentle Birth Choices.* Rochester, Vermont: Healing Arts Press, 1994.

Illich, Ivan. *Limits to Medicine: Medical Nemesis — the Expropriation of Health.* Harmondsworth, N.Y.: Penguin, 1977.

Kitzinger, Sheila. *Birth at Home.* Oxford and New York: Oxford University Press, 1979.

_____, ed. *The Midwife Challenge.* London: Pandora Press, 1988.

Kitzinger, Sheila, and Penny Simkin, eds. *Episiotomy and the Second Stage of Labour,* 2nd ed. Seattle, Washington: Pennypress, 1986.

Klaus, Marshall, John H. Kennell, and Phyllis H. Klaus. *Mothering the Mother.* Reading, Mass.: Addison-Wesley Publishing Co., 1993.

Klein, M.C. "Does Episiotomy Prevent Perineal Trauma and Pelvic Floor Relaxation?" Online *Journal of Current Clinical Trials,* Documents No. 10 and 20, July and September 1992. Montreal: Department of Family Medicine, McGill University.

Leavitt, Judith Walzer. *Brought to Bed: Childbearing in America, 1750-1950.* New York: Oxford University Press, 1986.

Liedloff, Jean. *The Continuum Concept: Allowing Human Nature to Work Successfully.* Reading, Mass.: Addison-Wesley, 1977.

Maize, Anessa. Sacred Birth Slide Presentation, Winnipeg, Manitoba, 1990.

Martens, Hildegard M. "The Relationship of Religious to Socio-Economic Divisions among the Mennonites of Dutch-Prussian-Russian Descent." Ph.D. dissertation, University of Toronto, 1977.

Martin, Emily. *The Woman in the Body: A Cultural Analysis of Reproduction.* Boston: Beacon Press, 1987.

Mason, Jutta. "Reflections on the Alternative Birth Culture." *The Birth Gazette* 5, no. 3 (1989).

_____. "The Meaning of Birth Stories." *The Birth Gazette* 6, no. 3 (1990).

Mitford, Jessica. *The American Way of Birth.* New York: Dutton Plume Books, 1993.

Noble, Elizabeth. *Childbirth with Insight.* Boston: Houghton Mifflin, 1983.

Odent, Michel. *Birth Reborn.* New York: Pantheon Books, Inc., 1984.

Peterson, Gayle. *Birthing Normally: A Personal Growth Approach to Childbirth,* 2nd ed. Berkeley California: Mindbody Press, 1984.

Rabuzzi, Kathryn Allen. *Mother with Child: Transformations through Childbirth.* Bloomington: Indiana University Press, 1994.

Redekop, Magdalene. "Still Life with Menno," *Canadian Literature*, no. 127 (winter 1990).

_____. *Mothers and Other Clowns: The Stories of Alice Munro*. London and New York: Routledge, 1992.

Rich, Adrienne. *Of Woman Born: Motherhood as Experience and Institution*. New York: Norton, 1986.

Rothman, Barbara Katz. *In Labor: Women and Power in the Birthplace*. New York, N.Y.: Norton, 1982.

Shuttle, Penelope, and Peter Redgrove. *The Wise Wound: Menstruation and Everywoman*. London: Harper Collins, 1986.

Silvera, Makeda. *Silenced: Talks with Working Class Caribbean Women,* 2nd ed. Toronto: Sister Vision, 1989.

Sosa, Roberto, John Kennell, Marshall Klaus, Steven Robertson, and Juan Urrutia. "The Effect of a Supportive Companion on Perinatal Problems, Length of Labor, and Mother-Infant Interaction." *The New England Journal of Medicine* 303, no. 11 (September 11, 1980).

Spallone, Patricia. *Beyond Conception, The New Politics of Conception*. Granby, Mass.: Bergin and Garvey, 1989.

Steinbeck, John. *The Grapes of Wrath*. New York: The Viking Press, 1967.

Swigart, Jane. *The Myth of the Bad Mother: The Emotional Realities of Mothering*. New York: Doubleday, 1991.

Turner, Joan, ed. *Living the Changes*. Winnipeg: University of Manitoba Press, 1990.

Urry, James. *None but Saints: The Transformation of Mennonite Life in Russia, 1789-1889*. Winnipeg: Hyperion Press, Ltd., 1989.

Walker, Barbara. *The Crone, Woman of Age, Wisdom, and Power*. San Francisco: Harper and Row, 1985.

Waring, Marilyn. *If Women Counted: A New Feminist Economics*. San Francisco: Harper, 1988.

Weed, Susun S. *Healing Wise*. Woodstock, N.Y.: Ash Tree Publishing, 1989.

_____. *Wise Woman Herbal for the Childbearing Year*. Woodstock, N.Y: Ash Tree Publishing, 1986.

Wertz, Richard W., and Dorothy C. Wertz. *Lying-In: A History of Childbirth in America*. New Haven: Yale University Press, 1989.